A Colour Atlas of
HYPERTENSION

Second Edition

Leonard M. Shapiro, MD, MRCP

Consultant Cardiologist
Papworth and Addenbrooke's Hospitals
Cambridge, England

Maurice B. Buchalter, MB, MRCP(I)

Clinical Lecturer
Department of Clinical Pharmacology
University of Cambridge
Honorary Senior Cardiac Registrar
Papworth Hospital
Cambridge, England

Wolfe Publishing Ltd

Published by Wolfe Publishing Ltd, 1991
Printed by BPCC Hazells Ltd, Aylesbury, Bucks, England
ISBN 0 7234 1637 0

A CIP catalogue record for this book is available from the British Library.

For full details of all Wolfe titles please write to Wolfe Publishing Ltd, Brook House, 2–16 Torrington Place, London WC1E 7LT, England.

Contents

Foreword

Physicians have long considered blood pressure to be one of the cardinal vital signs. In contemporary medicine, the importance of blood pressure is further heightened by the prominence of atherosclerotic disease as a leading cause of morbidity and mortality, the recognition that blood pressure is a powerful predictor of subsequent cardiovascular diseases, and the demonstration that treatment of hypertension lowers the risk of cardiovascular disease events. Reflecting over the last 30–40 years, the rôle of hypertension in clinical practice has rapidly escalated from one in which only a small number of patients with severe hypertension received medical attention to the current situation in which the evaluation and treatment of patients with mild to moderate hypertension is one of the most common responsibilities of the primary care physician. Indeed, management of patients with hypertension is the most frequent reason for outpatient visits to physicians in the United States.

In contrast to many clinical disorders, the causes of hypertension are many and its consequences are manifest in a wide variety of organ systems. This revised and expanded edition of the *Atlas* is an excellent collection of high quality photographs, x-rays, laboratory tracings and graphs which emphasize the systemic features of hypertension. The authors have wisely heeded the adage that "a picture is worth a thousand words". The associated text which compliments the pictorial material is succinct and easy to read. Truly, this is one of those books which has something for everyone. For medical students, it will serve as a useful introductory text which will not only stimulate their interest in hypertension but familiarize them with the diagnosis and pathophysiology of atherosclerotic cardiovascular disease in general. For practicing clinicians, the text will represent a handy reference with which to refresh their understanding and appreciation of hypertension and its consequences. The authors are to be congratulated on their revision of this unique and important text.

Professor Paul K. Whelton, M.D., M.Sc.
Director
Welch Center for Prevention,
Epidemiology and Clinical Research
The Johns Hopkins Medical Institutions

Preface to the second edition

Hypertension is one of the most frequently detected abnormalities in man. Depending on the criteria of definition, it has been found to affect up to 30% of the population. It causes detectable changes throughout the body, affecting not only the heart, but also the kidneys, the brain and the eye.

Many factors can give rise to hypertension, but even after thorough investigation a specific cause is found in only about 5% of cases. In these 'secondary' cases, endocrine, renal or other rare abnormalities are causative agents. A knowledge of the condition is therefore important to a wide range of clinical specialists. The authors have kept this in mind when preparing this extensively revised second edition. Indeed, *all* practising doctors dealing with hypertension – from generalist to specialist – will find much of value within these pages.

This Atlas deals with the investigative processes used with hypertensive patients and the pathological findings that commonly result in cases of both primary and secondary hypertension.

In this new edition there is a much expanded epidemiology section and a new section on clinical examination. The former demonstrates the relationship between hypertension and specific diseases and how the treatment of hypertension can prevent some diseases occurring.

As in the first edition, this Atlas does not deal with specific treatment regimens, but there is some reference to the non-pharmacological management of hypertension, as well as to the mechanisms of action of hypotensive drugs.

Preface to the first edition

Hypertension is the single most frequent disease in man, affecting up to 30% of the population. It is a multi-system disorder affecting the heart, kidney, brain and eye. In addition, rare endocrine disorders may present with hypertension. Hypertension is therefore of interest to any physician involved in clinical medicine.

This Atlas is designed to illustrate the important clinical causes and effects of hypertension. The book is largely based on pathology which is shown together with the results of clinical investigations.

In general we feel that all the topics are adequately covered. Obviously the selection must be personal, and our own interest in cardiology will be apparent. We have also included techniques that although not widely available at present may well become so in the future; for example, magnetic resonance and digital subtraction angiography.

It is hoped that this book will provide a better understanding of a common multi-system disorder.

Acknowledgements

We are indebted to the many friends and colleagues who contributed illustrations for this text. In particular we acknowledge the help of Sathia Thiru, who provided great help with the renal pathology, and Dr. Derek Appleton who helped with the renal radiology. Dr. Kim Fox, Dr. Nat Cary, Dr. Carole Warnes, Dr. Peter Crean, Dr. Owen Edwards, Dr. Adrian Dixon, Helen Murfit, Mr. Michael Michelli, Professor Morris Brown, and Mr. John Wallwork also kindly provided illustrations.

We wish to acknowledge the help of a number of hospital medical photography departments, including those at Addenbrooke's, Hinchingbrooke, National Heart, Dudley Road, Hammersmith, and Wythenshawe hospitals.

The authors are also grateful for permission to use pictures from other colour atlases already published by Wolfe Publishing Ltd.

Introduction and definition

In spite of major advances in the recognition and control of hypertension, raised blood pressure remains a major risk factor in the development of coronary artery, cerebrovascular and renal disease. Such diseases cause over half the deaths in western countries. The Framingham study demonstrated that the risk of developing coronary artery disease was twice as high in hypertensive as in normotensive subjects, and the risk of stroke was eight times higher.

Blood pressure varies throughout a 24-hour period, with a circadian rhythm. In addition, individuals exhibit swings in blood pressure related to physical activity or emotional stress. Therefore, the definition of hypertension can be difficult. A single blood pressure recording is not sufficient to diagnose mild hypertension, although in the presence of a severely raised blood pressure and other physical findings this may be adequate.

1

DEFINITION OF HYPERTENSION

A LEVEL OF BLOOD PRESSURE WHICH IS ASSOCIATED WITH INCREASED MORBIDITY AND MORTALITY AT SOME FUTURE TIME WHEN COMPARED WITH THE WHOLE POPULATION

1 The definition of hypertension is the level of blood pressure associated with an increased morbidity and mortality. This is unhelpful for identifying hypertension in an individual patient, but is useful for identifying the level at which a raised blood pressure becomes a risk for a population.

2

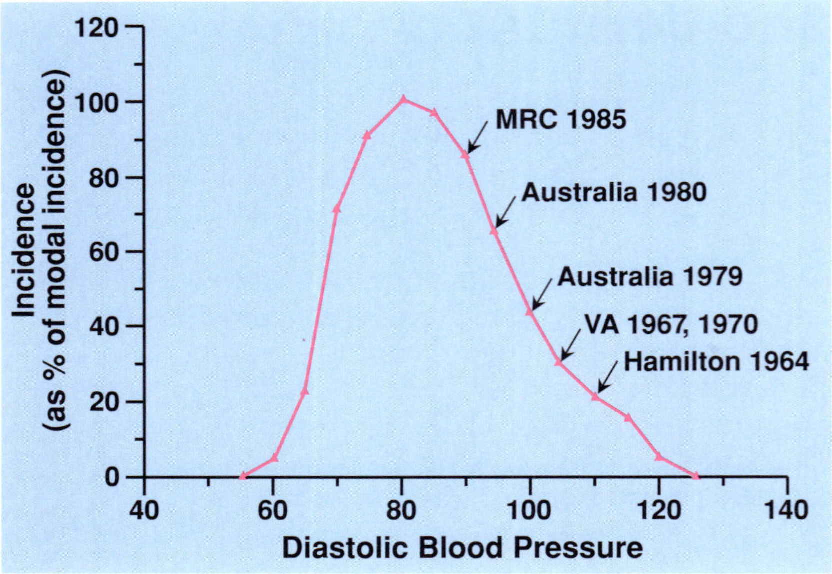

2 Approximately 5% of the middle-aged population of western countries have a diastolic blood pressure in excess of 110 mmHg, and a further 35% exceed 90 mmHg. These figures represent the distribution of diastolic pressures within an adult western population. The frequency distribution of diastolic blood pressure is not bimodal, and diastolic blood pressure is distributed as a continuous variable with positive skew. Therefore, the definition of the level at which systolic or diastolic blood pressure becomes elevated is very variable. The arrows represent various definitions of hypertension that were used for entry into the major hypertensive drug trials. As the century has progressed, blood pressure is being treated at a lower diastolic pressure.

Classification of hypertension

CLASSIFICATION OF HYPERTENSION BY AETIOLOGY			
I.	ESSENTIAL HYPERTENSION		
II.	SECONDARY HYPERTENSION		
	1.	RENAL	
		a.	Parenchymal
		b.	Renovascular
	2.	ENDOCRINE	
	3.	NEUROGENIC	
	4.	MECHANICAL	
	5.	EXOGENOUS	
	6.	MISCELLANEOUS	

3

3 Hypertension may be classified by aetiology. This divides hypertensive patients into those whose hypertension has no known cause (essential) and those whose hypertension is secondary to another disease process.

4

Causes of Hypertension

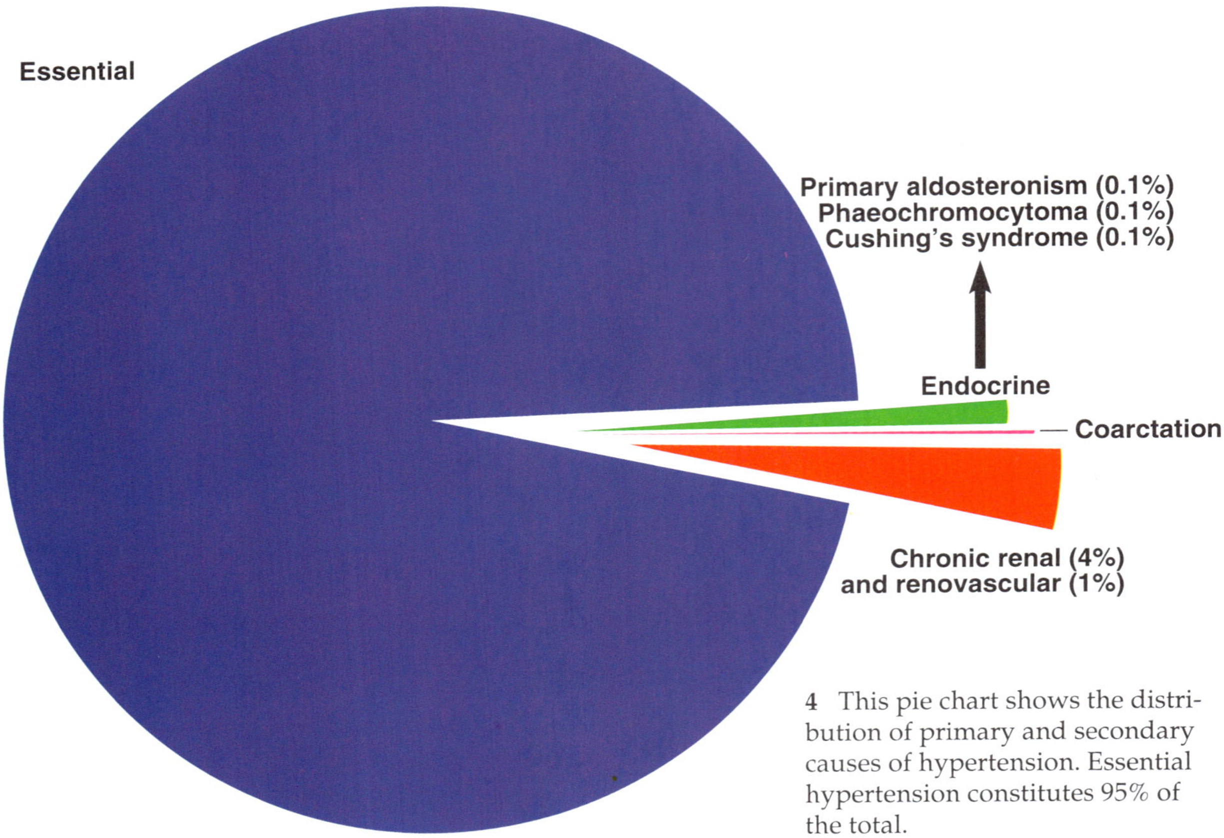

4 This pie chart shows the distribution of primary and secondary causes of hypertension. Essential hypertension constitutes 95% of the total.

5

RENAL CAUSES OF HYPERTENSION

I. PARENCHYMAL

a. Acute glomerulonephritis
b. Chronic nephritis, glomerulonephritis and pyelonephritis
c. Polycystic kidney
d. Hydronephrosis
e. Renin-producing tumour
f. Diabetic nephropathy

II. RENOVASCULAR

a. Fibromuscular arterial stenosis
b. Atherosclerotic arterial stenosis
c. Renal infarctions
d. Polyarteritis

6

ENDOCRINE CAUSES OF HYPERTENSION

I. ADRENAL

a. Phaeochromocytoma
b. Hyperaldosteronism (Conn's syndrome)
c. Cushing's syndrome
d. Congenital adrenal hyperplasia

II. PITUITARY

a. Acromegaly
b. Cushing's disease

III. ECTOPIC PRODUCTION OF HORMONES

a. Cortisol
b. Growth hormone
c. Catecholamines

7

MECHANICAL CAUSES OF HYPERTENSION

a. AV fistulae
b. Coarctation of the aorta
c. Aortic insufficiency – regurgitation
d. Atherosclerotic systolic hypertension

8

MISCELLANEOUS CAUSES OF HYPERTENSION

a. Toxaemia of pregnancy
b. Polycythaemia
  i. Rubra Vera
  ii. Gaisbock's syndrome
c. Carcinoid syndrome

5–10 The secondary causes of hypertension include those originating in the kidney and endocrine system, as well as mechanical causes, and other less common ones. The renal causes of hypertension can be divided into glomerular disorders, tubular–interstitial disorders, obstructive uropathy, vascular disorders, metabolic disorders, developmental abnormalities, tumours, and end-stage renal disease of any cause (**5**). The endocrine causes of hypertension include inappropriate hormone production from the adrenal and pituitary glands and ectopic sites (**6**). Coarctation of the aorta is the commonest mechanical cause of hypertension (**7**). In atherosclerotic elderly individuals, the systolic blood pressure may be considerably elevated. Arteriovenous (AV) fistulae and aortic regurgitation may lead to elevation of the systolic, but not the diastolic, pressure. There are a number of other causes of hypertension. Most of these are rare, but the use of oral contraceptives and hypertension associated with pregnancy are numerically the most common forms of secondary hypertension (**8–10**).

9

HYPERTENSION DUE TO EXOGENOUS SUBSTANCES

I. POISONING

a. Lead
b. Thallium

II. MEDICATION

a. Sympathetic amines
b. MAO inhibitors (combined with tyramine-rich foods)
c. Birth control pills
d. Prednisolone/Hydrocortisone

10

NEUROGENIC CAUSES OF HYPERTENSION

a. Respiratory acidosis
b. Brain neoplasm
c. Encephalitis
d. Acute porphyria

11

CLINICAL CLASSIFICATION OF HYPERTENSION

CLASS	BLOOD PRESSURE	FUNDOSCOPY	ECG	URINE
BORDERLINE	occasionally >90	N	N	N
MILD	140/90–160/105	N or GRADE I/II	N	N
MODERATE	140/90–160/105	N or GRADE I/II	LVH	ALBUMIN
	160/105–180/120	N or GRADE I/II	±LVH	±ALBUMIN
SEVERE	180/120+	N or GRADE I/II	±LVH	±ALBUMIN
MALIGNANT	Any level	GRADE III	±LVH	±ALBUMIN
	Any level	GRADE IV (Papilloedema)	±LVH	±ALBUMIN

11 The classification of the severity of hypertension is as difficult as its definition. The severity of hypertension relates not only to the level of blood pressure elevation, but also to the development of retinal, electrocardiographic, and renal changes. Classification of hypertension into borderline, mild, moderate, severe, and malignant allows a large overlap between the blood pressure levels in the subgroups. However, such classification does allow for a quantification of the level of target organ damage. Blood pressure levels are normally variable, as described above. The term labile, or borderline, is frequently used to describe diastolic pressures that only occasionally exceed 90 mmHg. Quite frequently, such borderline elevated blood pressures return to normal on a second, or subsequent, estimation.

The epidemiology of hypertension

Epidemiological studies have shown that there are two types of data available about arterial blood pressure. One concerns the long-term relationship between blood pressure and cardiovascular morbidity and mortality, and is dealt with in the next section. The second type relates to the predictors of blood pressure elevation. This includes the factors likely to determine the level of blood pressure reached by an individual within a population and to identify persons most likely to develop hypertension.

The frequency of hypertension within any population again depends on its definition. If a level of 140/90 is used, the prevalence doubles when compared with a blood pressure of 160/95. The effect of the level of blood pressure used to define hypertension is shown in **12**.

12

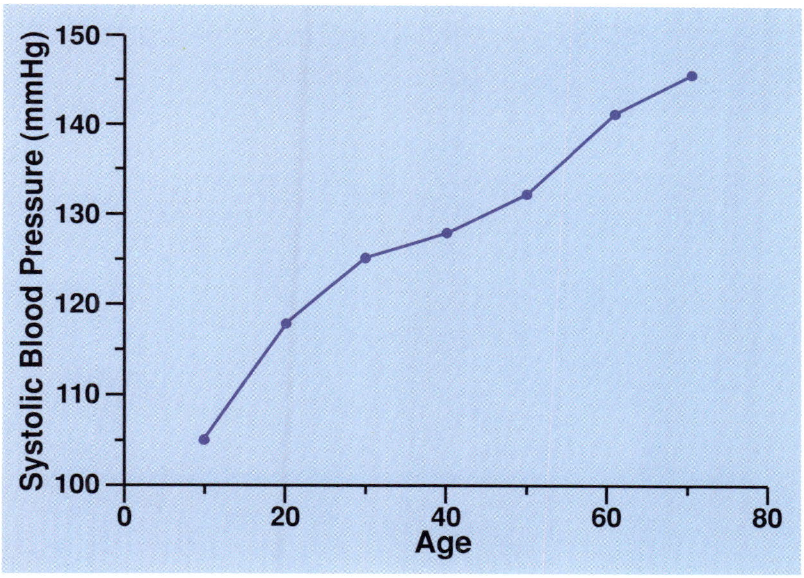

12 The relationship between systolic blood pressure and age in a western population. In western populations, systolic blood pressure rises with age, although this is not seen in certain pre-industrial societies.

13

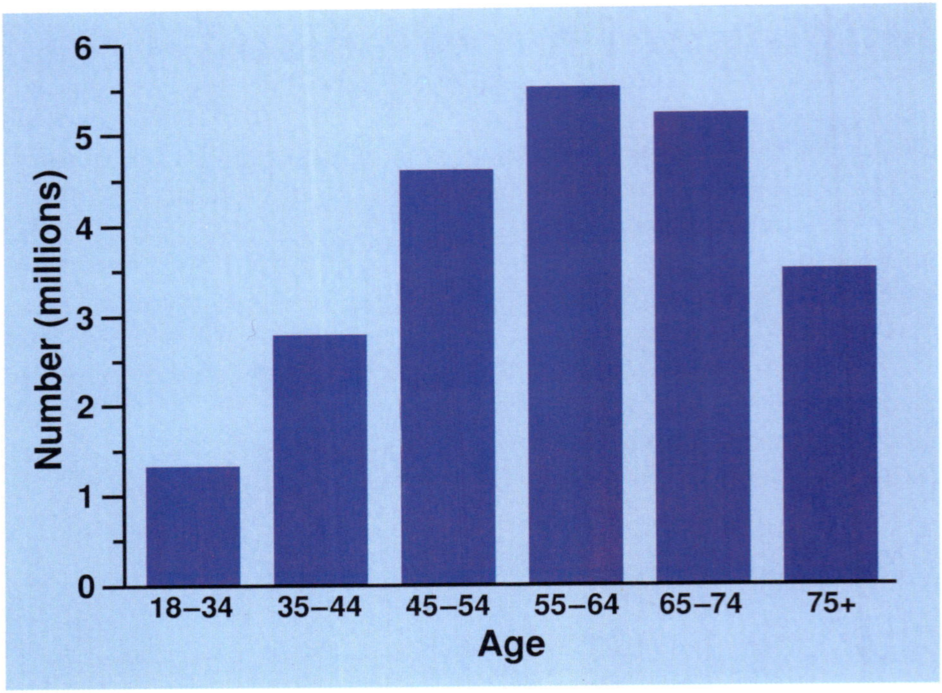

14

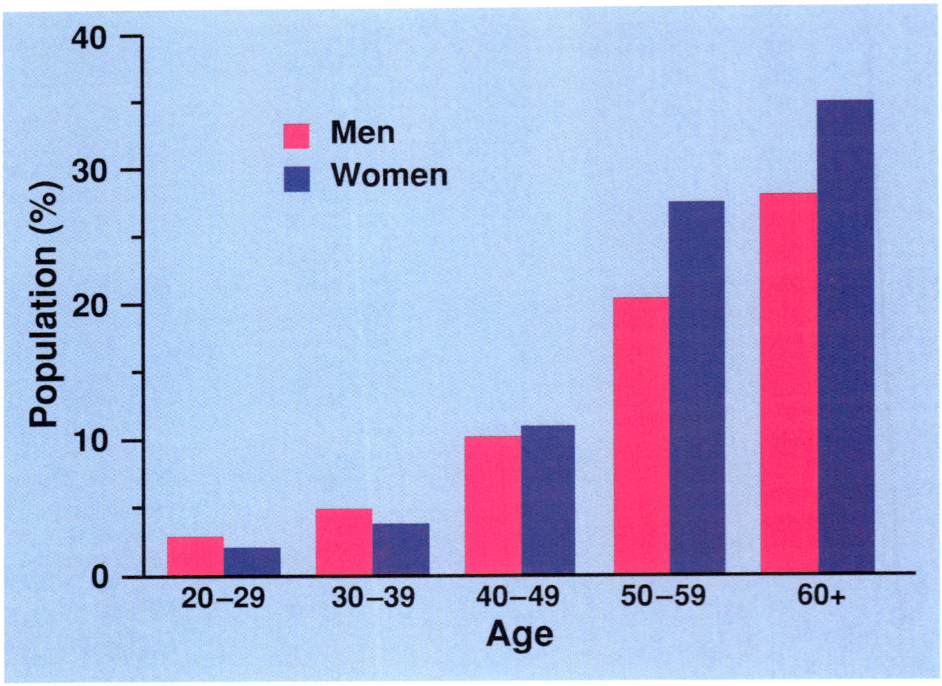

13, 14 These figures deal with the incidence of hypertension in the United States. The incidence of hypertension rises with age, reaching its peak in the 55–64-year-old age group (**13**). Hypertension is more common in men in the young and early middle-age groups, and more common in women in the older age groups (**14**).

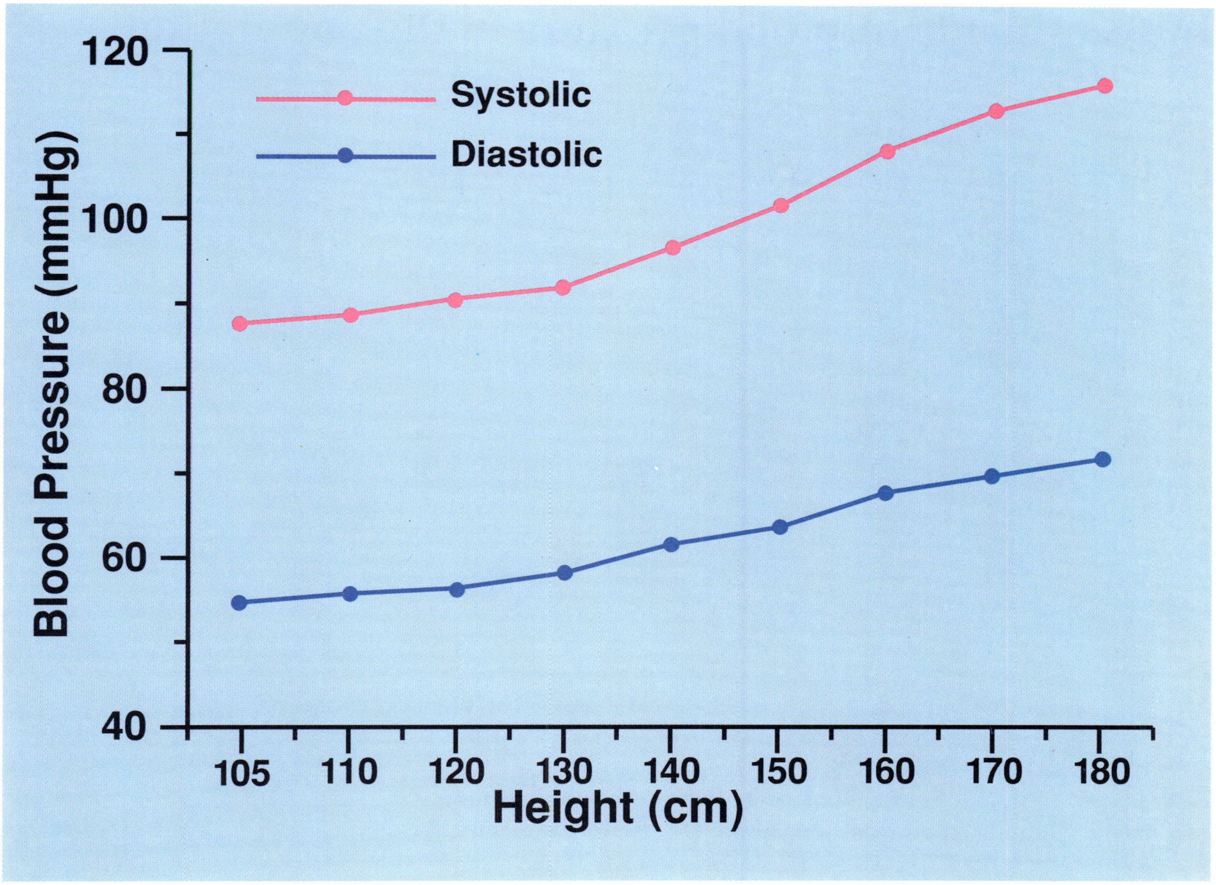

15 While the definition of hypertension in adults is difficult, extreme caution needs to be taken when diagnosing hypertension in children. Many children defined as hypertensive at one examination will be normotensive at a subsequent examination. In addition, there is no management policy for asymptomatic children. In normal children, however, blood pressure is related to height rather than to chronological age.

Determinants of blood pressure in the population

16

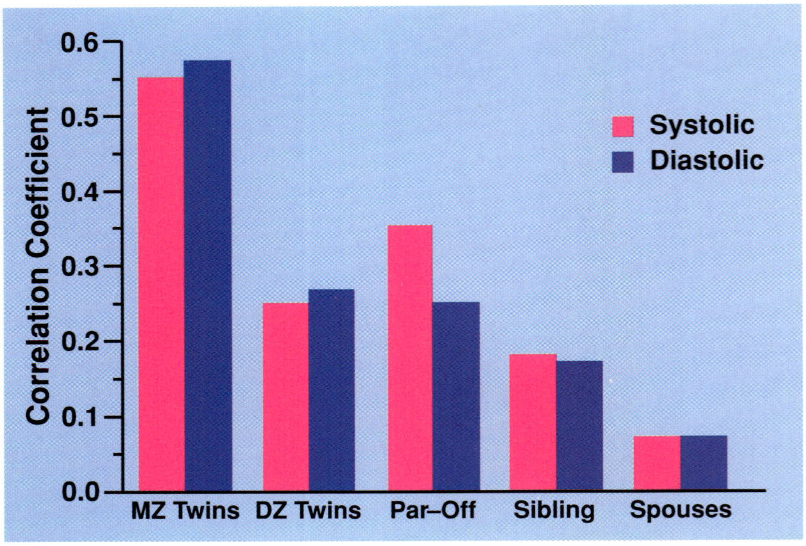

16 Hereditary factors are important in the development of hypertension. This figure demonstrates the incidence of hypertension in groups of relatives expressed as a correlation coefficient. Within pairs of monozygotic (MZ) twins, there is a high correlation of both systolic and diastolic hypertension. A similar relationship, though less strong, is observed between dizygotic (DZ) twins, between parents and their offspring (Par–Off), and between siblings. There is no association of hypertension in spouses. This evidence suggests that hereditary factors are important in the development of hypertension, and the stronger the relationship, the more likely that both individuals will be hypertensive. However, the correlation coefficient is not unity, and other non-hereditary factors must be important.

17

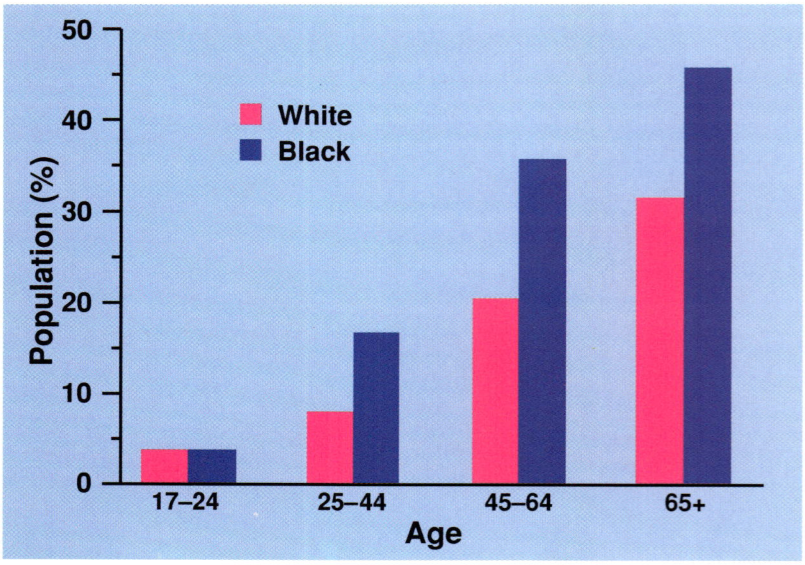

17 The incidence of hypertension among blacks is greater at every age beyond adolescence, and at any given level of blood pressure, the black population develops more vascular damage.

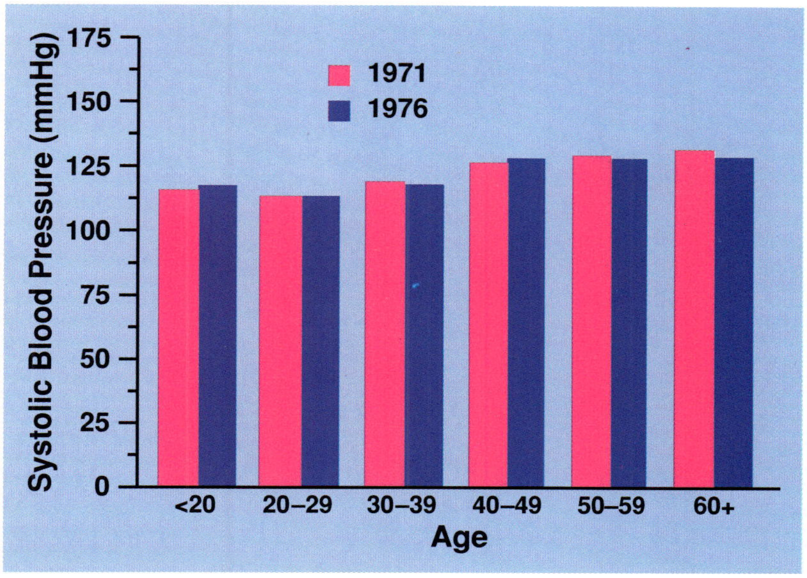

18

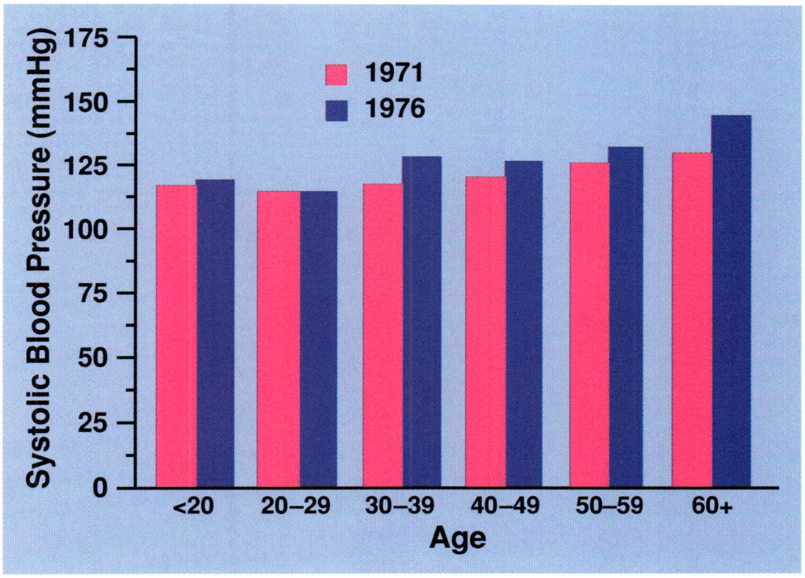

19

18, 19 The development of raised blood pressure is commonly seen in migrant populations compared to those who have remained in their indigenous surroundings. Comparison of blood pressure estimations in 1971 and 1976 in the Tokelans, a tribe in Polynesia, shows little difference in blood pressure when the population remained within its indigenous surroundings (**18**). However, in those Tokelans who migrated after 1971 into the urban areas of New Zealand, there had been a significant rise in blood pressure by 1976 (**19**). This would suggest that exogenous factors related to urban living are important in the development of hypertension.

20

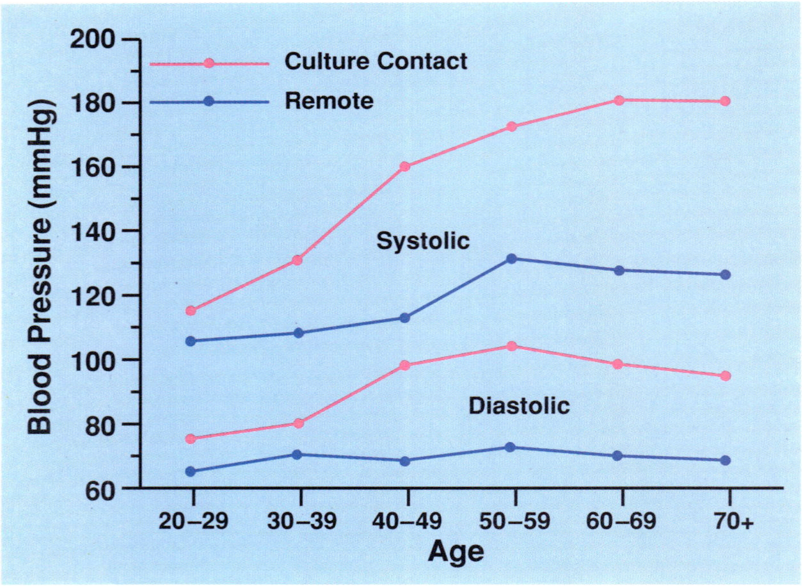

20 This figure compares the blood pressure in two Polynesian populations, one of which had a high degree of contact with western culture, and one that remained relatively isolated. There are clear differences in their blood pressures, particularly among the older age groups.

21

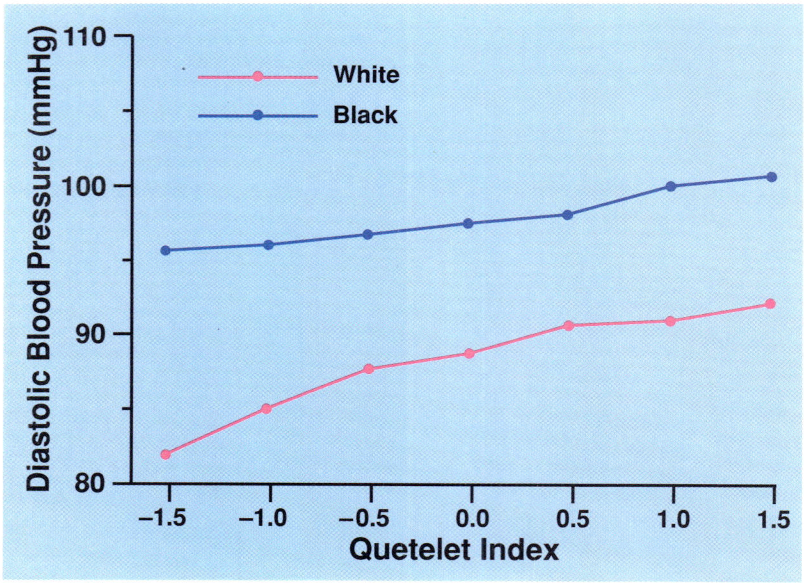

21 The mechanism by which body mass or obesity influences blood pressure is unknown. Studies suggest that it depends on general biological phenomena and is not greatly influenced by variations in genetic susceptibility. Insulin resistance may play a primary role in the relationship between blood pressure and obesity. The figure compares mean diastolic blood pressure in Evans County residents, aged 35–59 in 1960, with a standardized Quetelet index. This index is a relationship of height and weight, which standardises weight according to height. A consistent relationship of blood pressure to body mass exists, which is probably independent of other blood pressure determinants. This mechanism is poorly understood, but maintenance of ideal body weight often reduces the risk of hypertension, whereas weight gain markedly increases it.

22 The influence of social class appears to be important in the development of hypertension. This figure, showing the incidence of hypertension among different social classes, demonstrates the lower risk in administrative staff compared with professional, clerical and others. It would thus appear that those with the highest social class have the least risk of developing hypertension.

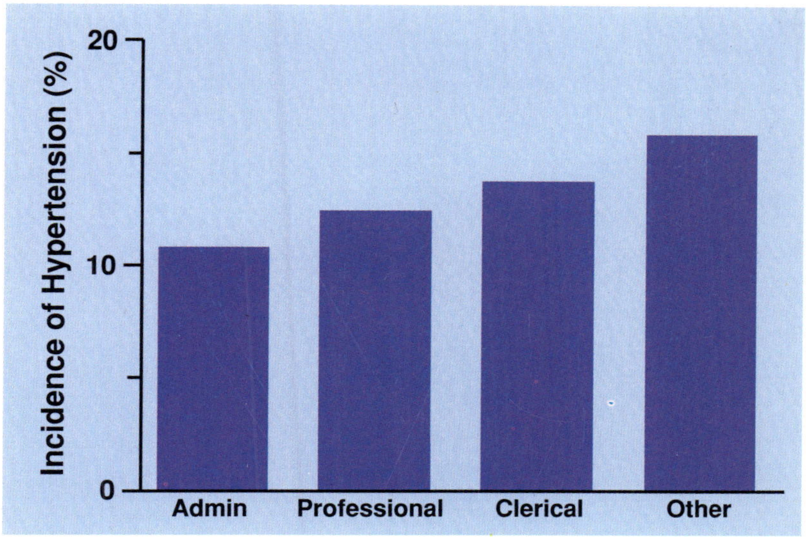

22

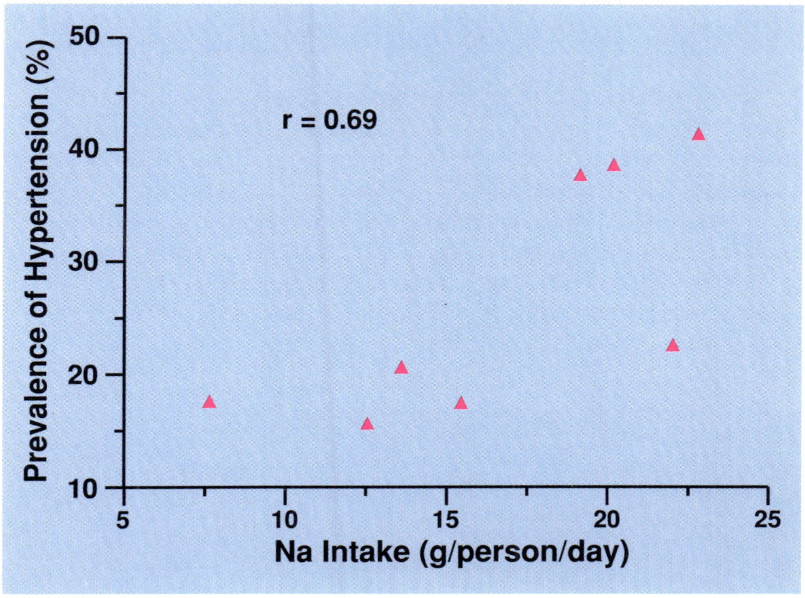

23

23 Excess intake of sodium chloride in the diet may be important in the pathogenesis of hypertension. If so, sodium restriction could be valuable in the prevention and treatment of hypertension. The evidence is suggestive of this link, but not conclusive. Possibly, subgroups of individuals with a family history of hypertension are at greater risk of the hypertensive effect of excessive salt intake. Other data, however, have rather conflicted with this hypothesis. This figure compares sodium chloride intake with prevalence of hypertension in several Japanese towns. It would appear from this evidence that there is a relationship between sodium intake and the prevalence of hypertension in large populations.

24

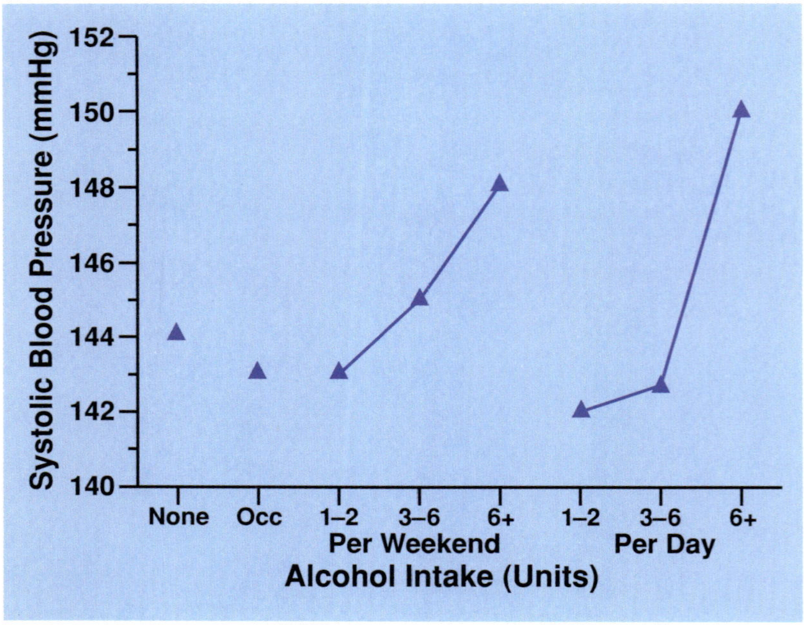

24 There is a clear association between alcohol consumption and hypertension. Consumption of as little as 30–40 g per day may be sufficient to produce hypertension, but its hypertensive effect disappears within a few days of abstinence. The aetiology of alcohol-related hypertension remains obscure; however, chronic alcohol ingestion can be associated with excess secretion of cortisol and can mimic Cushing's syndrome. The British Regional Heart Study demonstrates that systolic blood pressure rises with the number of alcohol units consumed, on either a weekend or a daily basis.

25

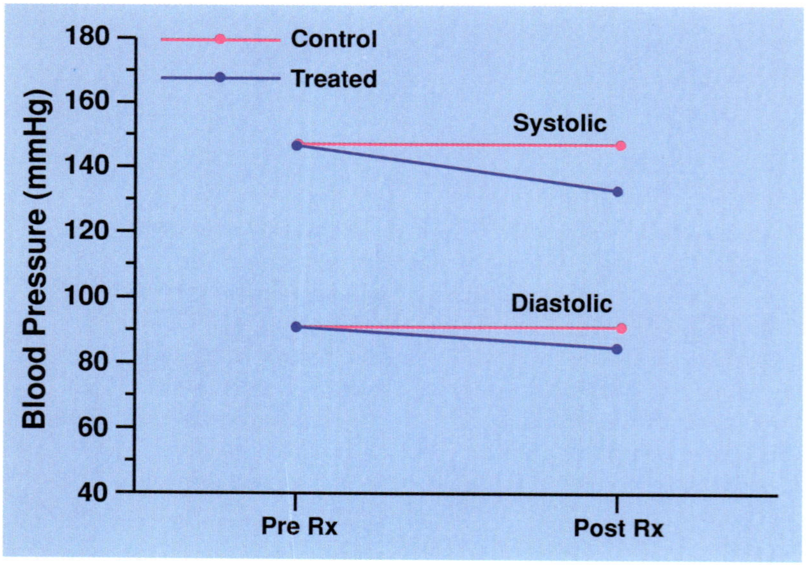

25 The effect of stress on blood pressure and the development of hypertension remains unclear. However, in this study, a relaxation technique (Rx) has been shown to have a significant effect on reducing both systolic and diastolic pressure.

Risk and consequences of raised blood pressure

The higher the level of blood pressure, the greater the likelihood of the premature development of various complications due to the acceleration of atherosclerosis and cerebral haemorrhage. If untreated, approximately half of hypertensive patients die from cardiovascular disease, a third from stroke, and 10–15% from renal disease. The more rapidly accelerating the hypertension, the more frequently death is due to renal failure.

26

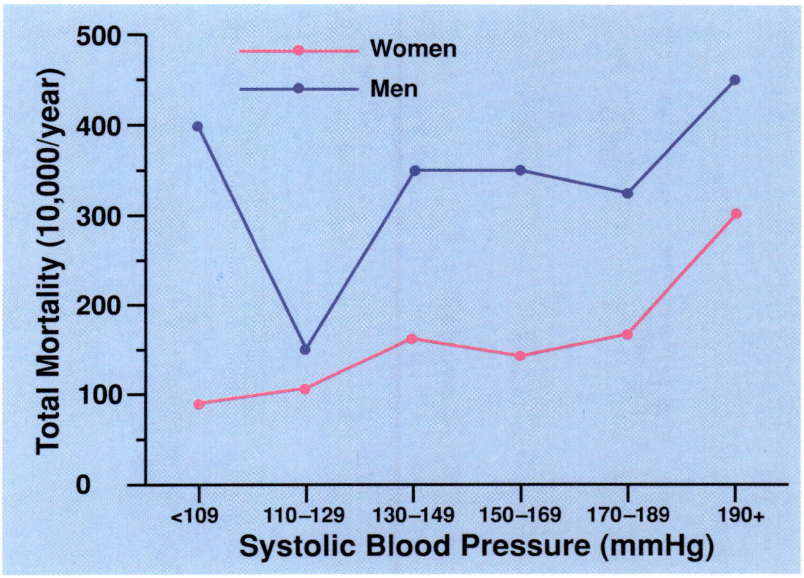

26 Total mortality, as shown on the y-axis, increases in both men and women as systolic blood pressure rises. It may be noted that low blood pressure carries a poor prognosis in men, probably because of the association with heart failure.

27

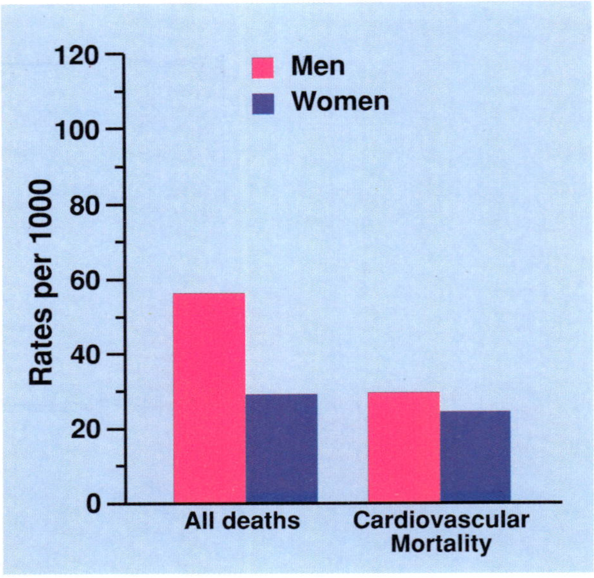

27 Systolic blood pressure is closely related to the development of the complications of hypertension. The development of cardiovascular disease accounts for the majority of all deaths in the hypertensive population.

28

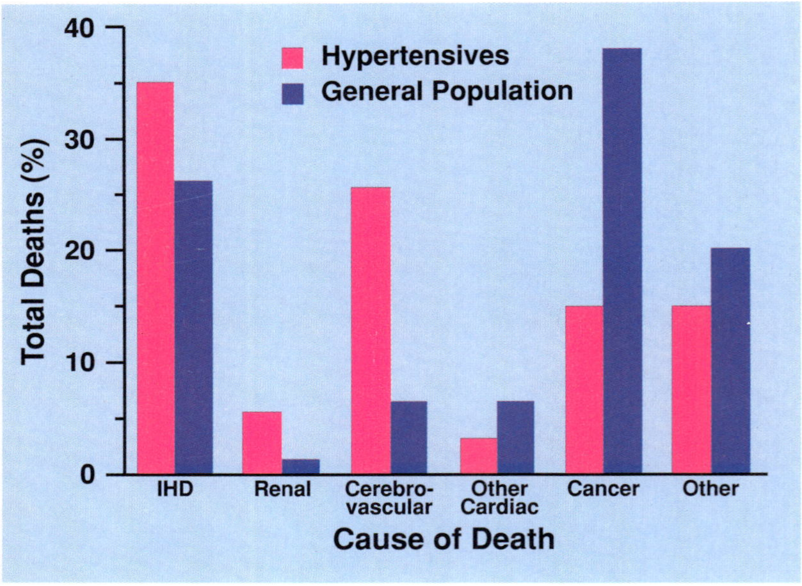

28 The causes of this increased mortality are accelerated atherosclerosis, ischaemic heart disease (IHD), and cerebrovascular disease, and an increased incidence of renal failure. Malignant deaths (i.e. cancer-related) feature less in hypertensives because of premature vascular and renal deaths.

29 The Framingham study shows that in both men and women the incidence of coronary artery disease increases with the degree of hypertension. Normotensive individuals have approximately half the risk of those definitely hypertensive, and those with borderline hypertension have an incidence of coronary disease midway between these two levels.

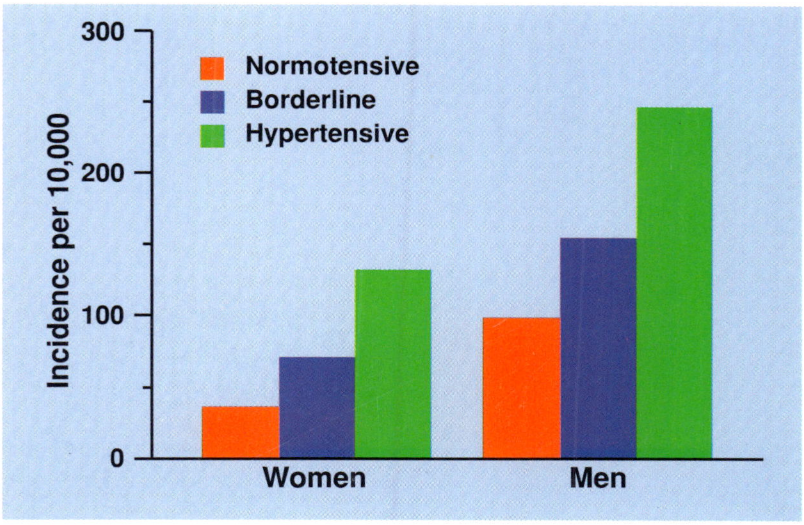

29

30, 31 It may be noted that this increased risk of ischaemic heart disease over a 24-year period is seen through all age ranges, both in men (**30**) and women (**31**).

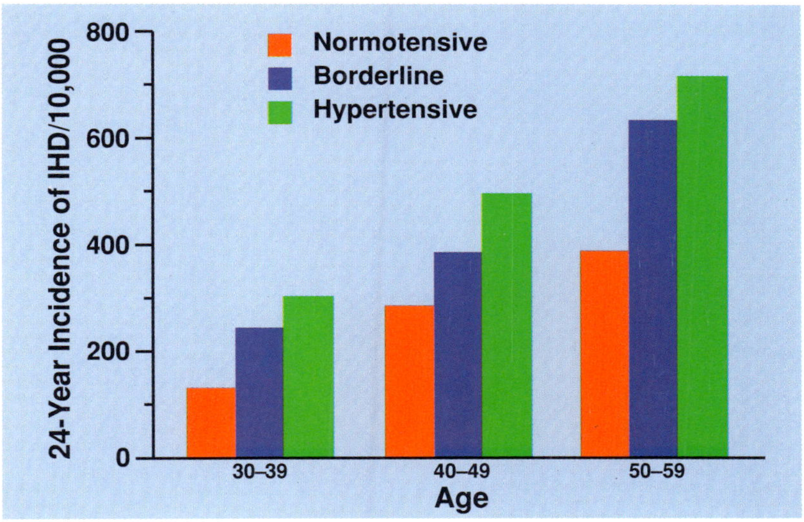

30

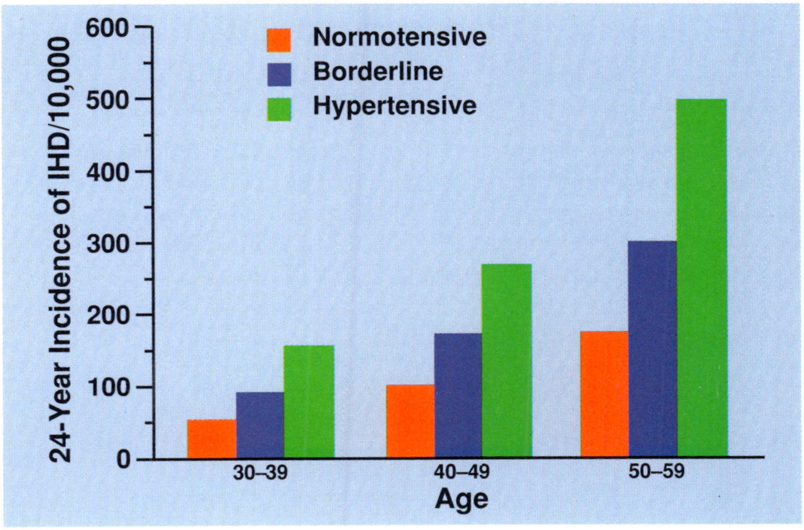

31

32

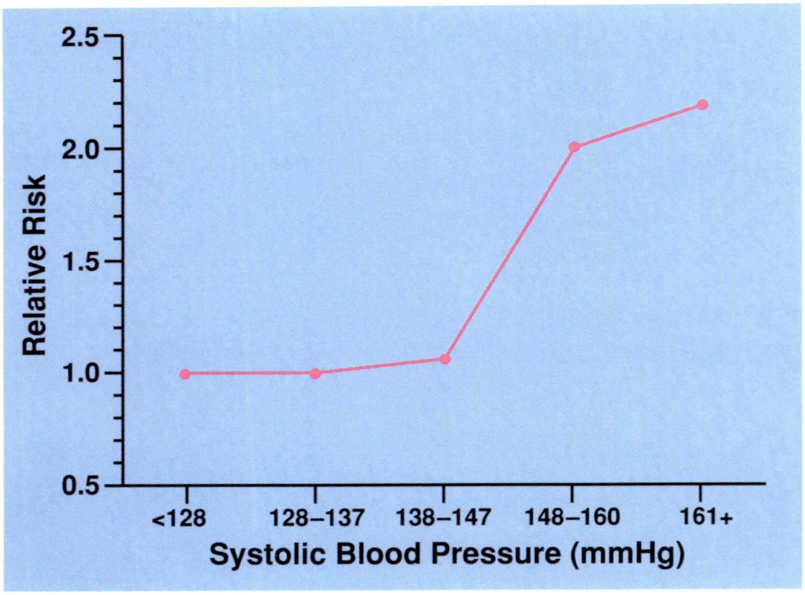

33

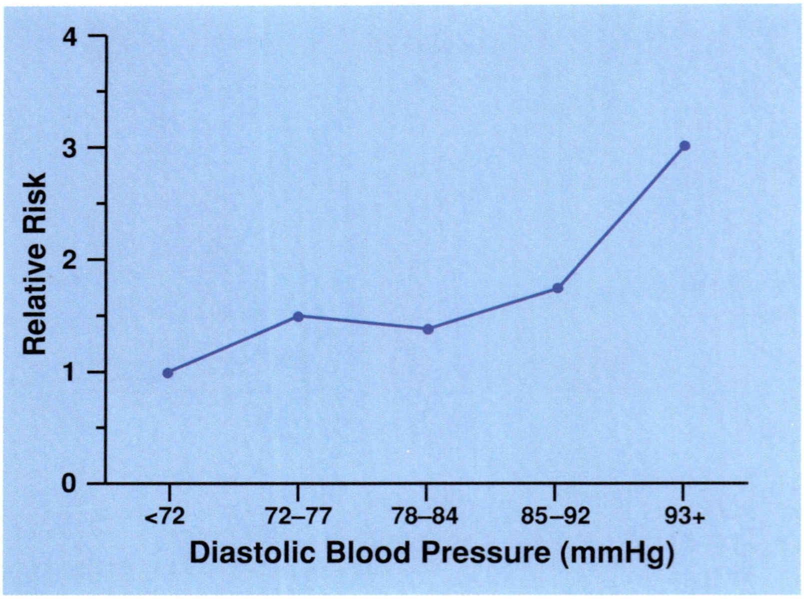

32, 33 The relative risk of developing coronary artery disease is related to increasing systolic and diastolic blood pressures. For systolic blood pressures below 138–147 mmHg, the relative risk remains approximately unity. Thereafter, small increases in blood pressure result in a rapidly increasing risk of developing ischaemic heart disease (**32**). A similar increase in relative risk is seen with elevation of the diastolic blood pressure (**33**).

34–36 The Framingham study has estimated the incidence per 10,000 population of the major complications of hypertension. In all, complications are more common in men than women, and hypertensive individuals have a greatly increased risk of congestive heart failure (**34**), intermittent claudication (**35**), and cerebral infarction (**36**). Individuals with borderline hypertension have intermediate levels of risk.

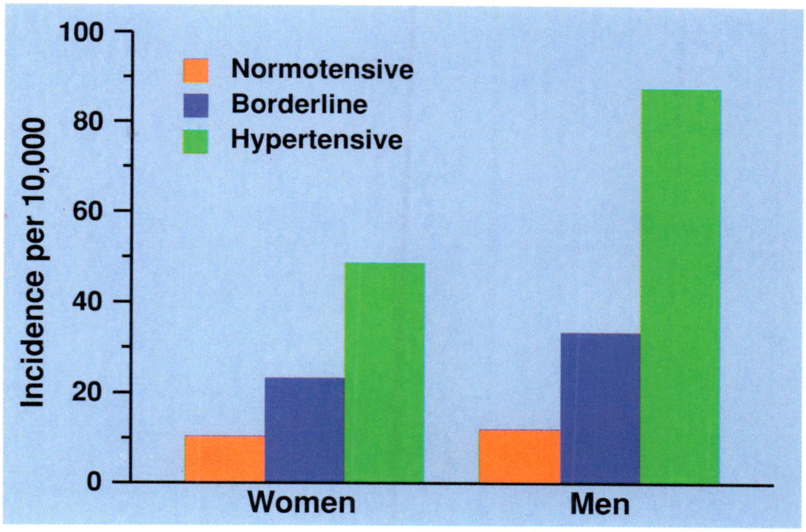

34

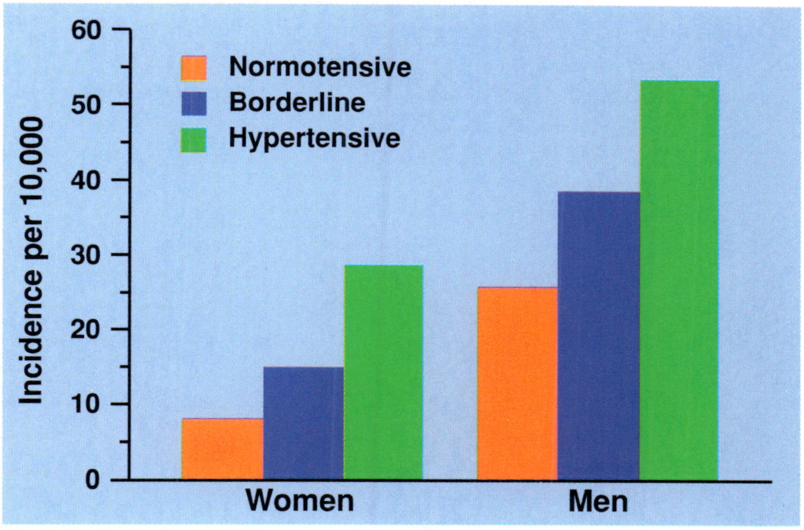

35

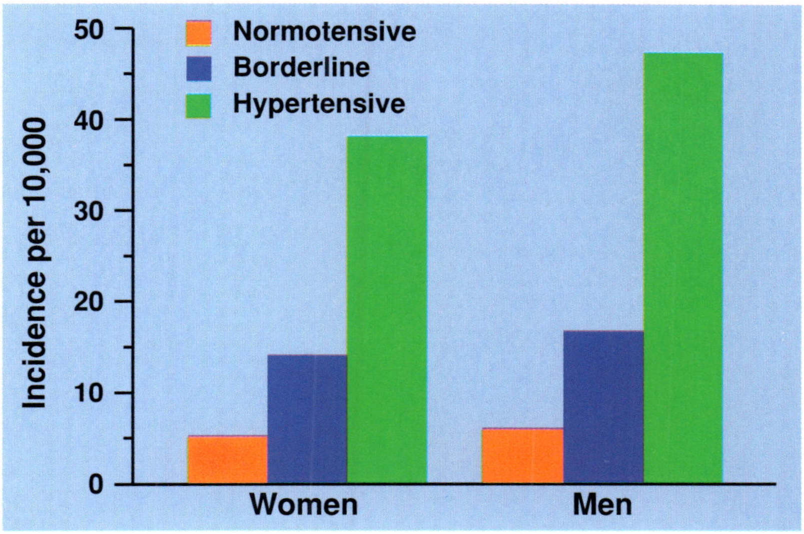

36

37

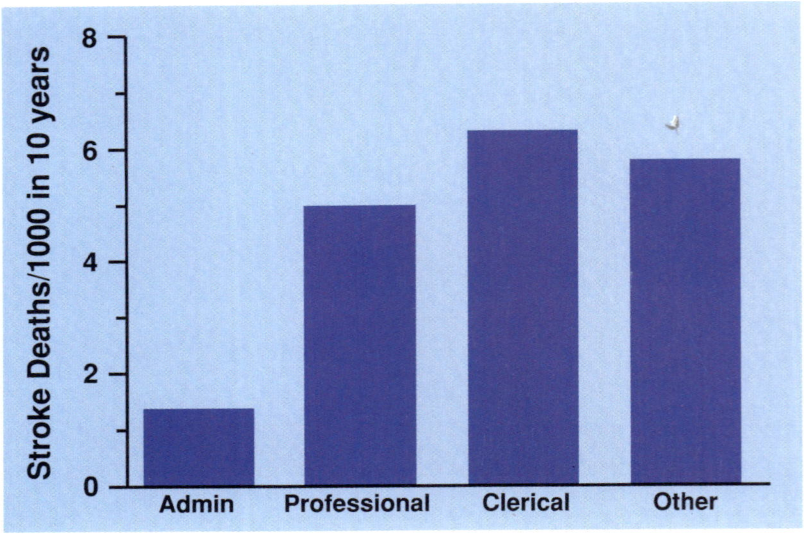

37 The Whitehall study compared the risk of stroke with social class and found the risk was lowest among administrative staff, and higher within the other professional and non-professional groups. Compare this with the incidence of hypertension in these groups shown in the section on the determinates of blood pressure in the population (**22**).

38

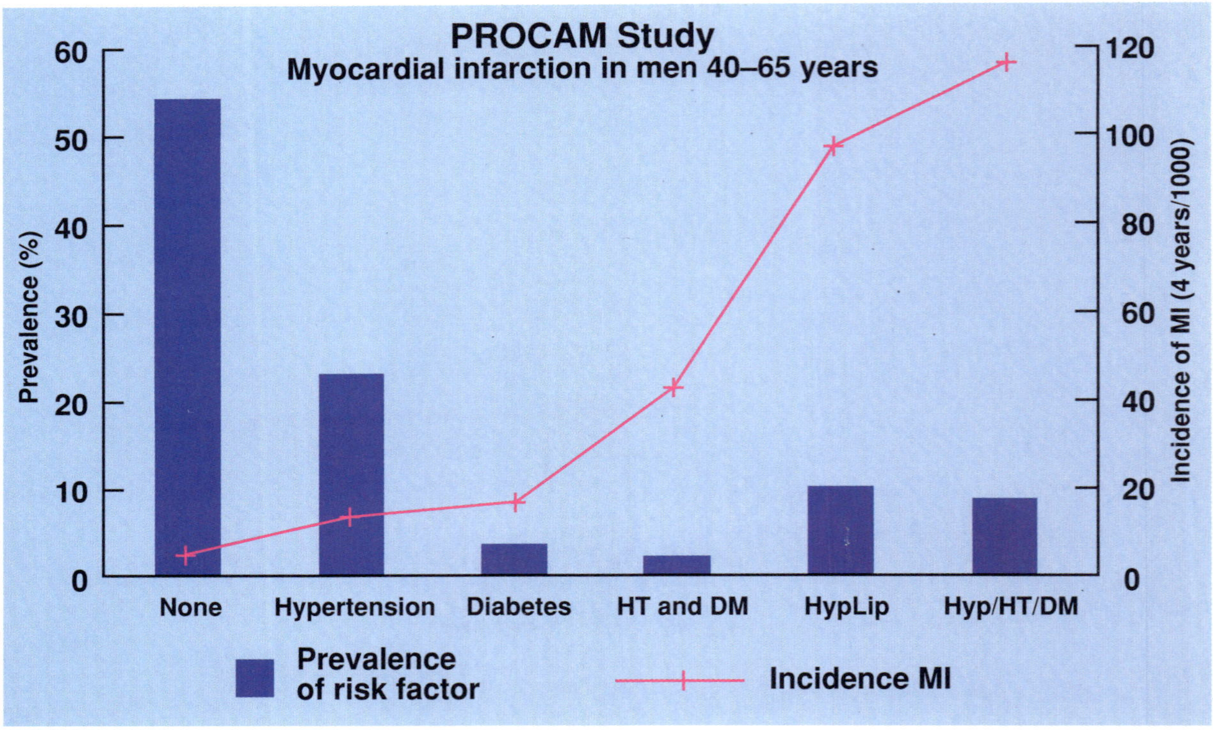

38 The PROCAM study showed the prevalence of various risk factors among men aged 40–65 years who developed a myocardial infarction. The majority of patients who develop a myocardial infarction (MI) have no obvious risk factors. Hypertension (HT) is statistically the most common risk factor in those developing myocardial infarction, and while the risk of developing myocardial infarction is very great in those who are hypertensive, hyperlipidaemic (HypLip, Hyp) and have diabetes (DM), they are numerically a small group.

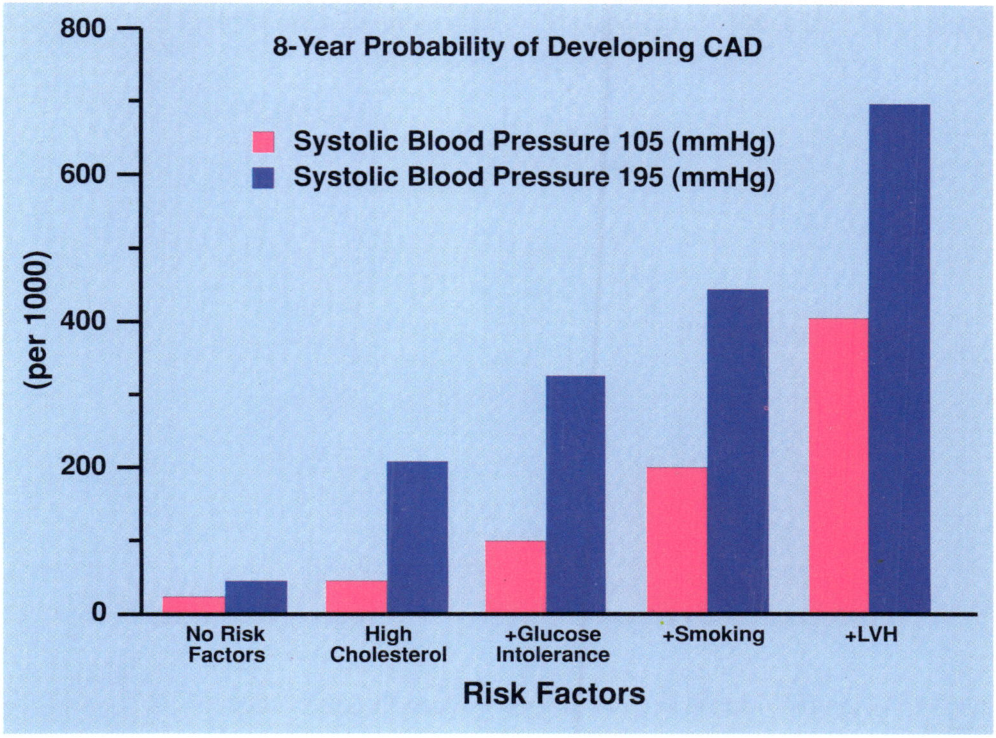

39 Hypertension interacts with the other major risk factors for coronary artery disease (CAD), hyperlipidaemia and cigarette smoking, and their combined effects are more than additive. This data from the Framingham study shows the risk of a 40-year-old man developing cardiovascular disease over an eight-year period. Increasing levels of systolic blood pressure are shown in relation to other risk factors. Individuals with normal blood cholesterol (185 mg/100 ml) and no other risk factors of heart disease show little increase in the probability of developing heart disease with rising blood pressure. However, a similar 40-year-old man with hyperlipidaemia and other risk factors has a considerably increased probability of developing coronary disease. In summary, there is only a 4% risk of coronary disease associated with hypertension when no other risk factors are present, but with a similar increase in blood pressure in the presence of hyperlipidaemia, glucose intolerance, cigarette smoking, and ECG abnormalities, there is a 70% risk of coronary disease developing in the eight-year period.

Effects of anti-hypertensive treatment

40

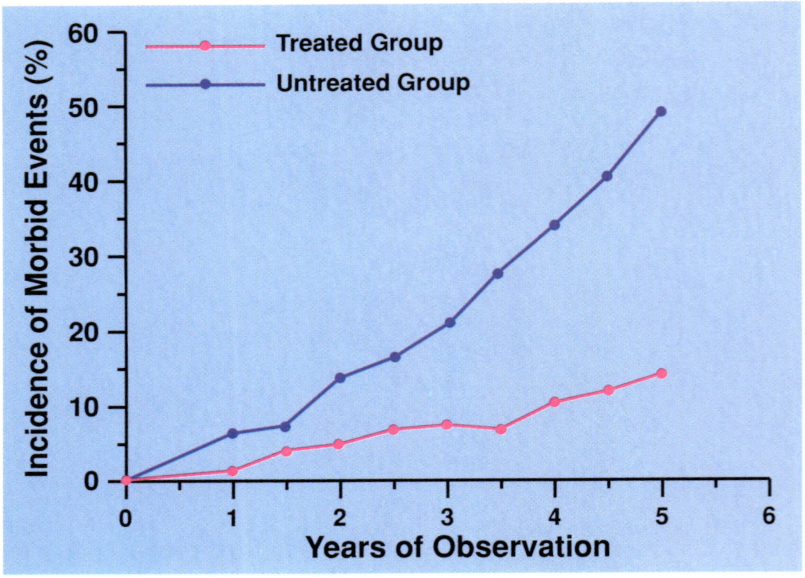

40 The Veterans' Administration Co-operative Study, published in 1970, shows the incidence of morbid events against the number of years of observation in treated and untreated hypertensive patients. At five years, the differences are considerable, with only 15% of treated hypertensives having suffered a morbid event, whereas in excess of 50% of those untreated had done so.

41–43 The effect of treatment of severely hypertensive patients compared to untreated individuals is shown in a series of multi-centre studies. The incidence of vascular deaths (**41**), the development of coronary heart disease (CHD, **42**), and the development of stroke (**43**) are shown. The Hypertension Detection and Follow-up Programme III (HDFP III), the European Working Party on Hypertension in the Elderly (EWPHE), and the Study in General Practice of Coope and Warrender (COOPE), all show a significant reduction in the incidence of vascular deaths with the treatment of severe hypertension. A cumulative total for these and other studies also shows a significant reduction. A similar overall reduction is shown in the incidence of coronary heart disease (**42**). A strong association is seen between the reduction in the incidence of stroke and the treatment of severe hypertension (**43**).

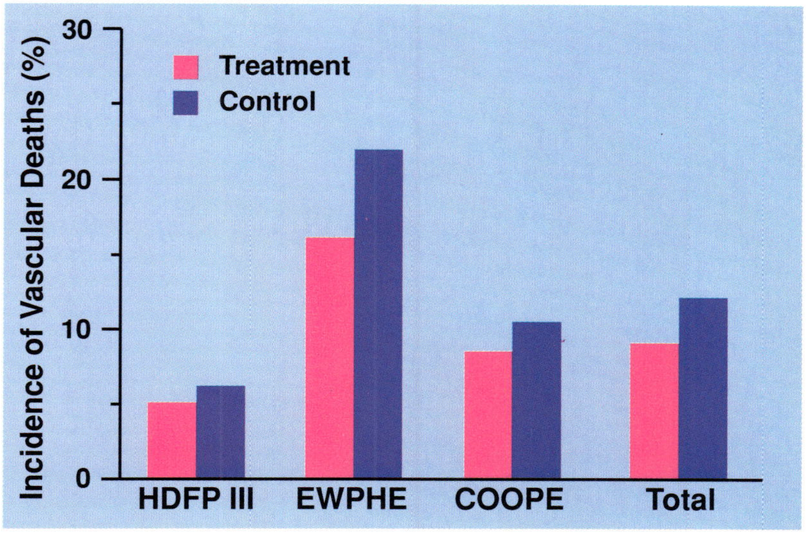

41

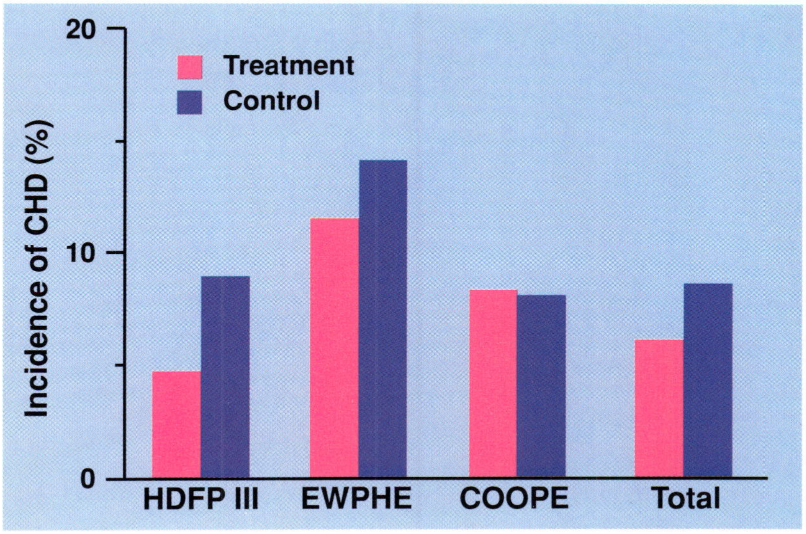

42

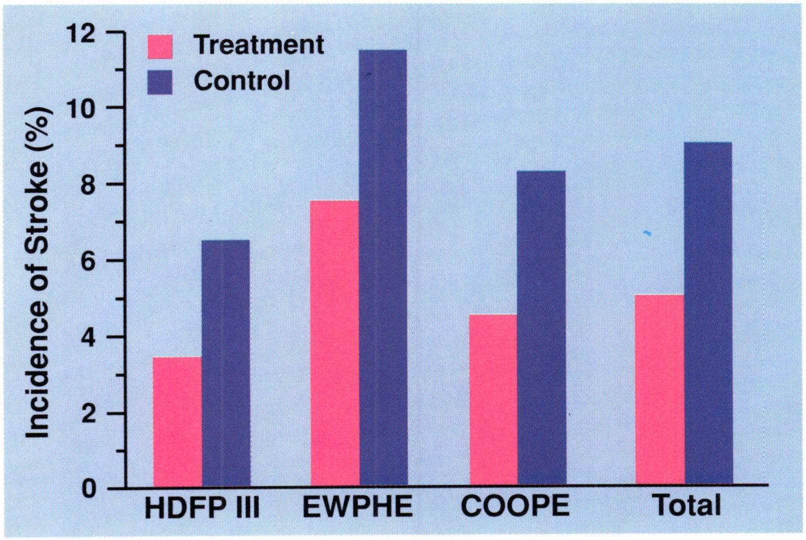

43

44

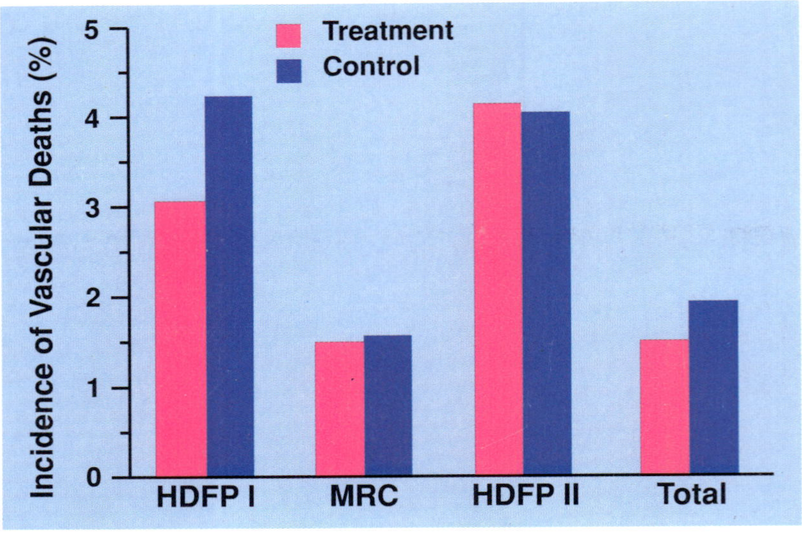

45

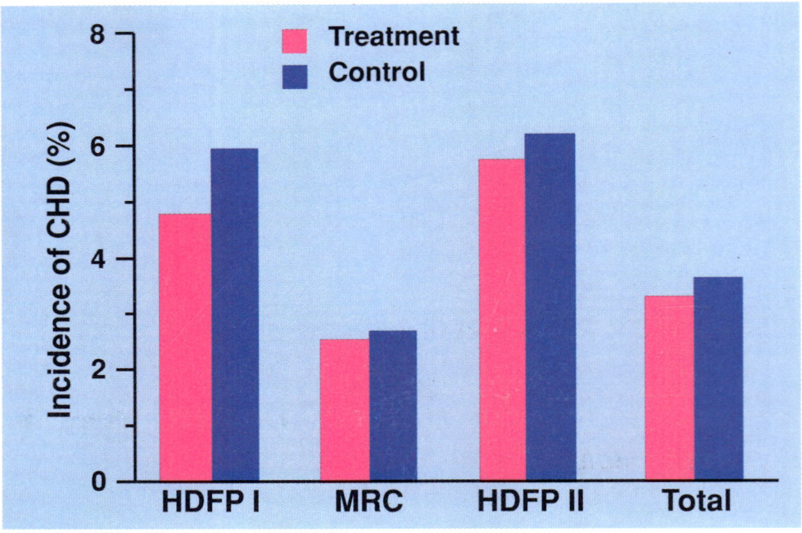

46

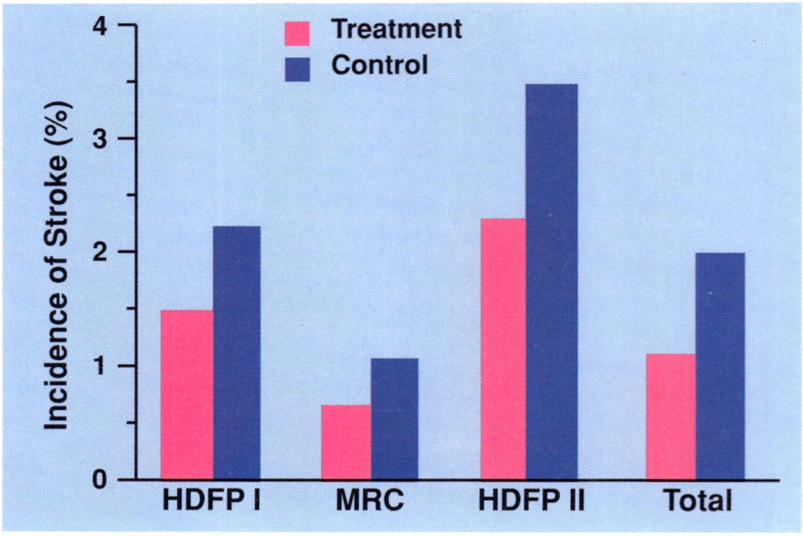

44–46 Treatment of mild hypertension is a more contentious issue and similar multicentre studies have more equivocal results on the reduction of vascular deaths and coronary heart disease. However, the reduction in the incidence of stroke remains important. **44, 45** demonstrate that, of the various studies, including the Hypertension Detection and Follow-up Programme I and II (HDFP I and HDFP II) and the Medical Research Council Trial (MRC), only the HDFP I shows a reduction in vascular deaths and the incidence of coronary disease. A cumulative meta-analysis of all the studies available for vascular death and development of coronary artery disease suggests there is a reduction in the incidence of these conditions with treatment. However, this effect is smaller than one might expect on the basis of blood pressure as a risk factor for common artery disease (**44, 45**). In comparison, there is a strong reduction in the incidence of stroke with the treatment of mild hypertension (**46**).

Clinical evaluation of hypertensive patients

Other than the measurement of the arterial blood pressure, the history and examination of a hypertensive patient are often unrewarding. Even the measurement of the blood pressure may be difficult, as the patient's blood pressure may vary throughout the day and is dependent on many factors. The goals of patient assessment should include assessing the cause of hypertension, its severity, and the degree of end-organ damage.

7a

GOALS OF PATIENT ASSESSMENT

1) Assess the cause of the hypertension
2) Assess the severity of the hypertension
3) Assess the degree of end-organ damage

47b

HISTORY

1) Symptoms of any causes of secondary hypertension (pages 40–96)
2) Symptoms of the effects of hypertension (pages 97–142)
3) Family history of hypertension
4) Family history of the causes of hypertension
5) Symptoms of associated disorders

47 In the history, we may elicit the symptoms related to, and a family history of, the causes and effects of hypertension and associated disorders.

48

EXAMINATION

1) Signs of the causes of secondary hypertension (pages 40–96)
2) Signs of the effects of hypertension (pages 97–142)
3) Measurement of blood pressure

49

BASELINE INVESTIGATIONS

1) Urea, creatinine and electrolytes
2) Urinalysis
3) Chest radiograph
4) Electrocardiogram

48 When examining a patient with hypertension, one must measure the blood pressure and also attempt to elicit signs of the causes or effects of hypertension.

49 While it is possible to undertake a large number of investigations in a hypertensive patient, those listed are regarded by many as the baseline investigation required in all hypertensives.

Measurement of the blood pressure

50

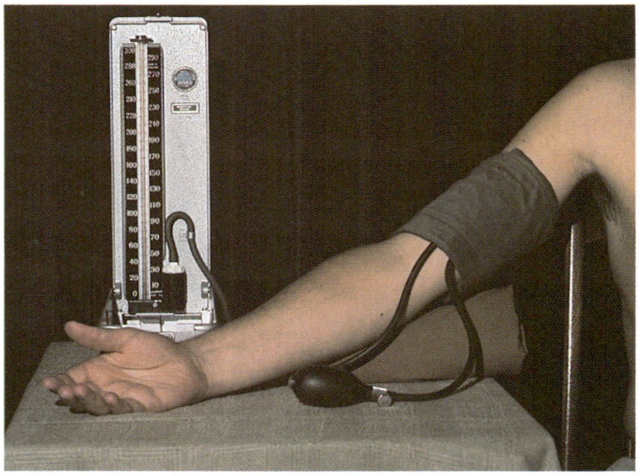

50 Correct measurement of the blood pressure requires an appropriate cuff size, correct positioning of the bladder, and that the patient should be seated or lying comfortably relaxed, with the arm straight or slightly flexed at heart level, and with the arm being supported. A mercury manometer is generally more accurate than an aneroid type, which needs annual calibration.

51

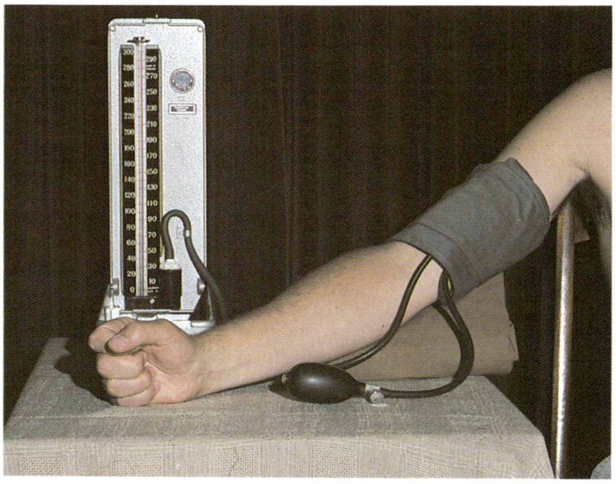

52

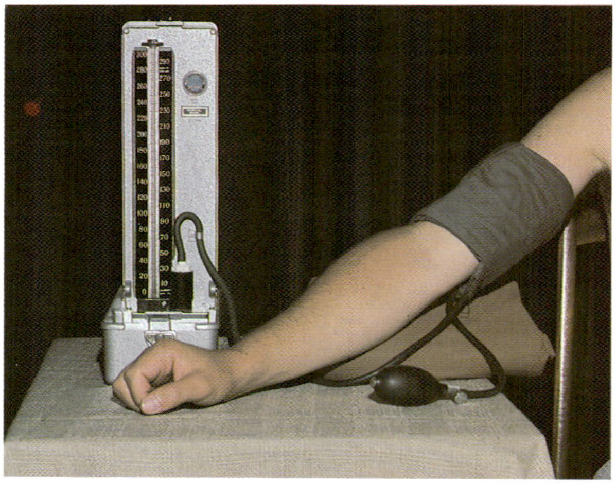

51–57 The following figures demonstrate some of the errors that can occur in a measurement of blood pressure. While the cuff and bladder are correctly positioned, and the arm is supported by a pillow, this patient has a clenched fist, which may artificially raise the blood pressure (**51**). If the bladder is not centred over the brachial artery, an inaccurate measure of blood pressure will occur (**52**). If the cuff is not wrapped snugly around the upper arm, it may fall before it can be inflated over the brachial artery, and thus make correct identification of the Korotkoff sounds difficult (**53**). Careless wrapping of the cuff around the arm may allow the bladder to escape during inflation. This prevents the pressure in the bladder from being transmitted accurately to the arm (**54**). The cuff must be directly in contact with the skin, and the arm straight or almost so, to allow accurate measurement of blood pressure (**55**). The size of the cuff is important and its width should

53

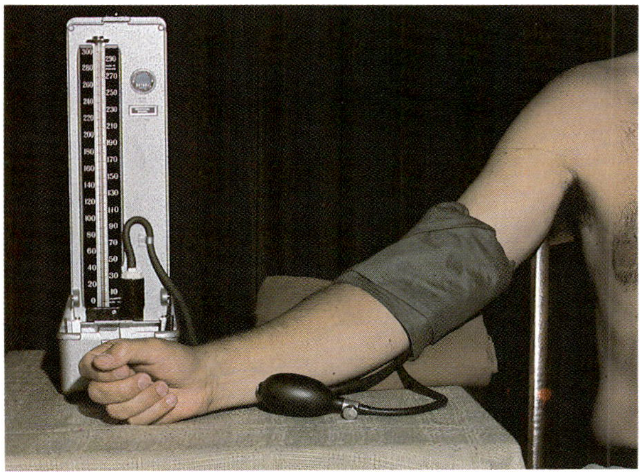

54

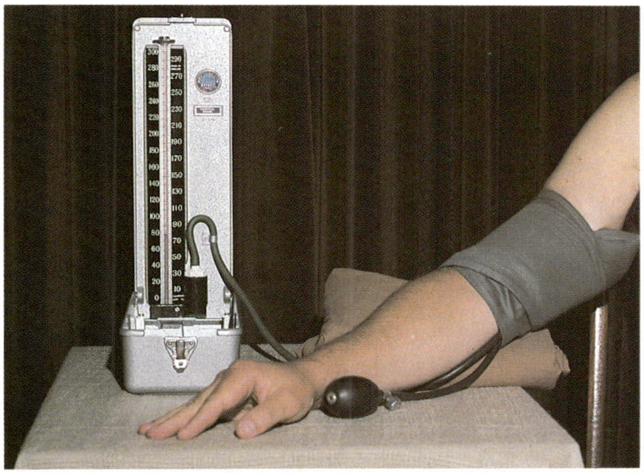

55

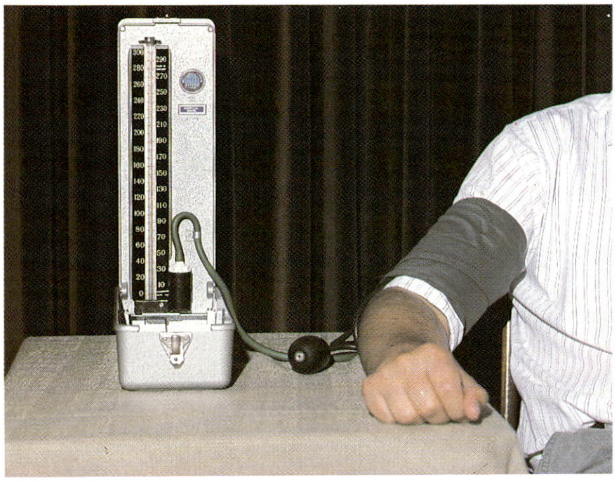

56

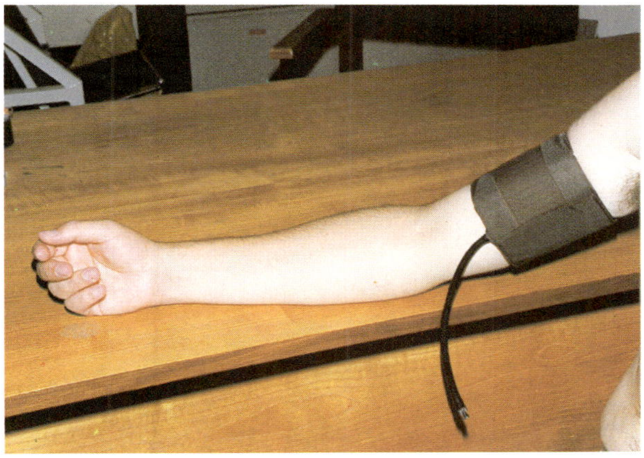

57

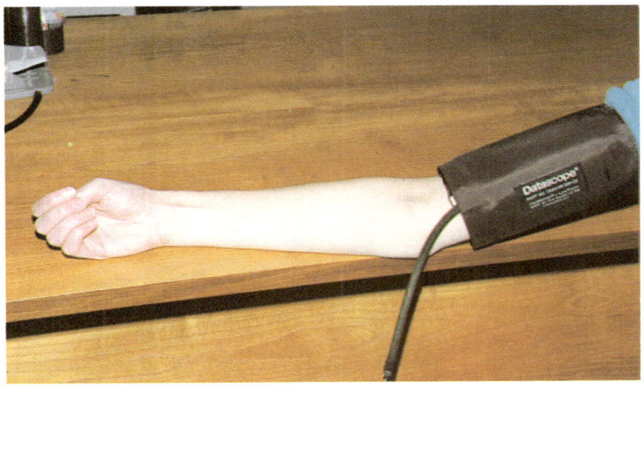

be at least 40% of the circumference of the limb. The standard five-inch cuff is designed for adults with an arm of average size. If a cuff is applied to a large upper arm or a normal adult thigh, arterial pressure will be overestimated. This may lead in turn to spurious hypertension in the obese. When a standard cuff is applied to a small arm, pressure will be underestimated. These figures demonstrate inappropriately small (**56**) and large (**57**) cuffs applied to a standard sized arm.

58

KOROTKOFF SOUNDS

I. Abrupt sharp sound as pressure is reduced to just below systolic

II. Prolonged louder murmuring sound

III. Good clear sound with only a slight murmur

IV. Abrupt muffling of sounds

V. Disappearance of sounds

58 The cuff should be inflated rapidly to approximately 30 mmHg above the anticipated systolic blood pressure. The cuff is then slowly deflated, and auscultation with the stethoscope bell is used to detect the Korotkoff sounds. The Korotkoff sounds are shown, and while phase V represents the diastolic blood pressure, it is good clinical practice to record both phase IV and phase V. If the blood pressure is elevated, it is preferable to allow the patient to remain in a quiet room and repeat the measurements later. Some clinicians measure the blood pressure three or more times over a period of 20–30 minutes. They then record the mean pressure for these recordings. Whichever technique is used, it is important that any clinician employs a standard technique for measuring and recording blood pressure.

59

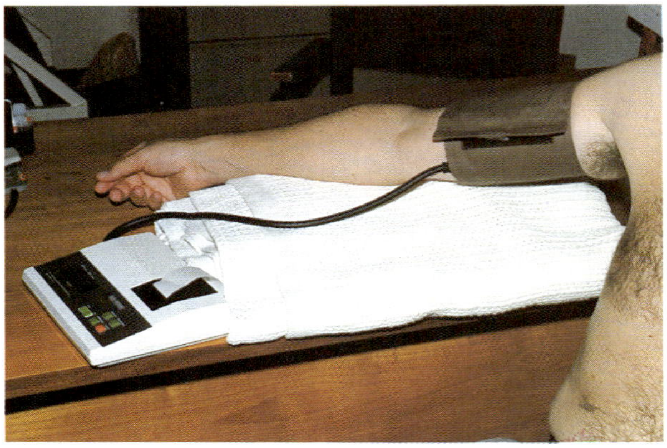

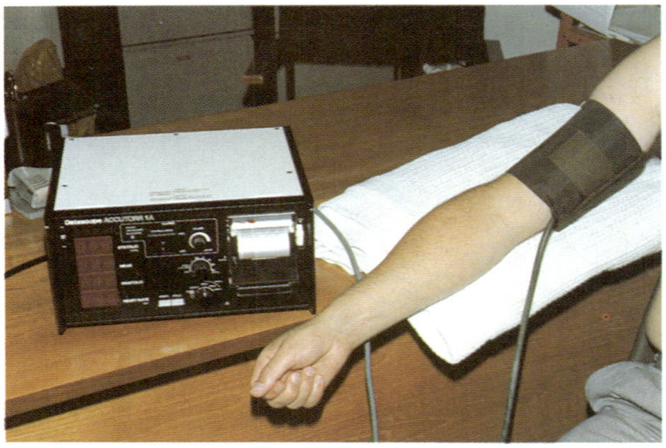

60

61

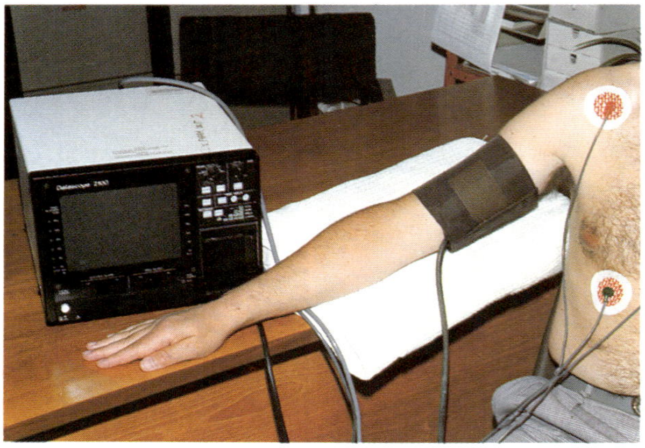

59–61 Measurements of the blood pressure can become automated or semi-automated. Using a variety of ultrasound and auscultatory-based techniques, blood pressure can be measured either as a single reading (**59**), on a continuous-paper recording (**60**), or continuously with the electrocardiogram (**61**). The latter is, of course, useful in coronary care settings.

62

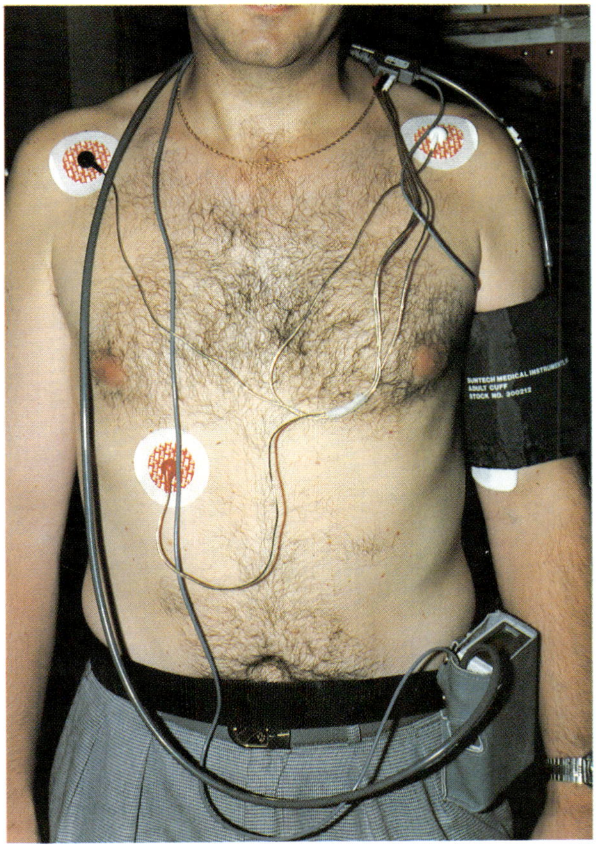

63

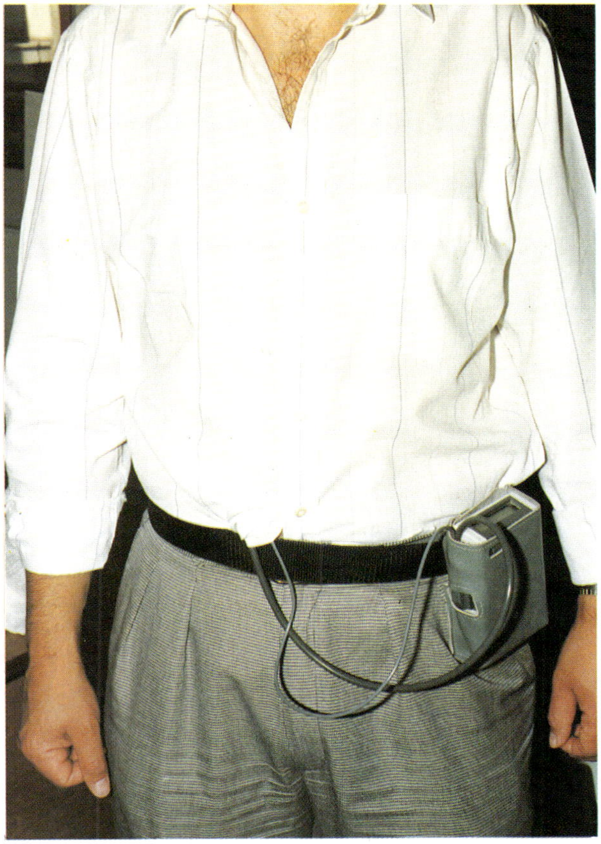

62–63 There are a number of devices that allow the ambulatory recording of blood pressure. These may be invasive, or use techniques similar to those described in the previous figures. Here we see a patient equipped for ambulatory blood pressure and electrocardiographic recording (**62**). The device fits neatly beneath normal clothing and hangs from a belt from the waist (**63**).

64

RENAL AND VASCULAR

i) Age under 30 years
ii) Diastolic blood pressure greater than 120 mmHg
iii) Continuous bruit in the epigastrium or flanks
iv) Accelerated hypertension
v) History of flank pain, haematuria or renal trauma
vi) Palpable kidney
vii) Hypertension resistant to treatment

PHAEOCHROMOCYTOMA

65

i) Unusual lability of blood pressure
ii) Symptomatic paroxysms of hypertension
iii) Spells of — Pallor
— Palpitation
— Perspiration
— Headache
iv) Hypertensive reaction to general anaesthetic or anti-hypertensive drugs

66

COARCTATION OF THE AORTA

i) Diminished and/or delayed femoral pulses
ii) Rib notching on chest radiograph

67

CONN'S SYNDROME

i) Serum potassium less than 3.6 mmol/l
ii) Urinary potassium greater than 30 mmol/24 h in the absence of diuretic therapy

68

CLINICAL SIGNS OF

i) Cushing's syndrome
ii) Acromegaly

64–68 There are a number of features in the history and physical examination that would suggest the presence of a secondary cause of hypertension. These causes include renal and renovascular disease (**64**), phaeochromocytoma (**65**), coarctation of the aorta (**66**), and Conn's syndrome (**67**). The physical examination of a patient with Cushing's syndrome and acromegaly may reveal the presence of hypertension (**68**).

Causes of hypertension

While there are many different causes of hypertension originating in many different organ systems, most patients have no known cause for their raised blood pressure.

Essential hypertension

69

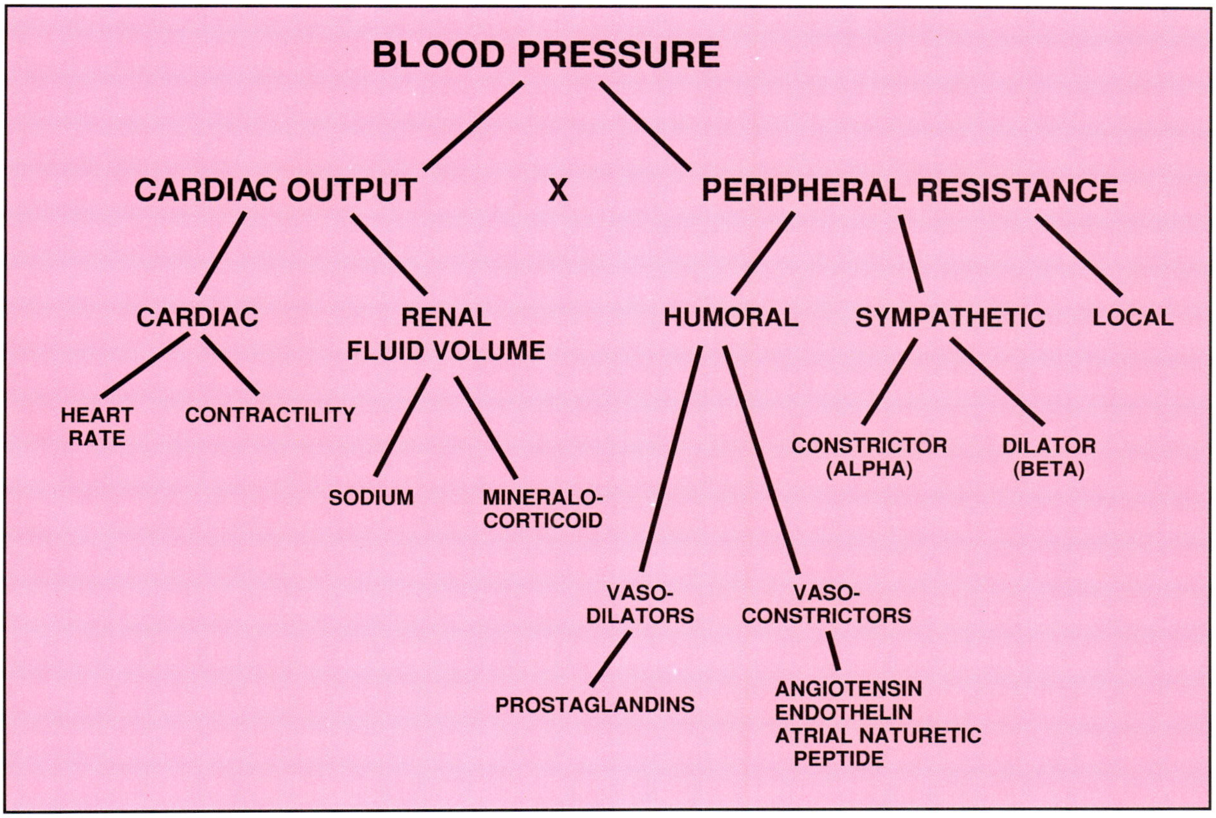

69 A diagrammatic representation of some of the factors involved in the control of blood pressure. These factors control cardiac output, fluid volume (both intra- and extra-vascular), and blood vessel calibre and responsiveness. None of these factors are independent and few are normal in hypertensive patients. However, while there are many theories, the causes of essential hypertension are poorly understood.

Secondary hypertension

To establish the diagnosis of essential hypertension, a secondary cause has to be excluded. Such cases constitute a small proportion of all patients with hypertension, but may be apparent clinically or on simple investigation. The most important causes are renal, endocrine, and vascular.

Secondary causes of hypertension

Renal causes

After the use of oral contraceptives, renal disease is the most common secondary cause of hypertension. In unselected adult populations, up to 2–4% of hypertensives will have renal disease as the aetiological factor. Hypertension usually appears late in the course of renal disease, and contributes further to the deterioration of renal function. Renal disorders that may lead to hypertension may be classified into glomerular, tubular interstitial, and vascular disorders, each subdivided as below.

Glomerular disorders

Acute proliferative glomerulonephritis
Post-infectious glomerulonephritis, anti-glomerular basement membrane disease (Goodpasture's syndrome), lupus nephritis, mesangio capillary glomerulonephritis, focal proliferative glomerulonephritis.

Chronic glomerulonephritis
This is the end-stage of any form of glomerulonephritis.

Tubular interstitial disorders

Primary
Acute pyelonephritis, focal segmental glomerulosclerosis (FSGS), reflux nephropathy (sometimes referred to as chronic pyelonephritis, tubulo-interstitial nephritis (allergic, toxic and infectious), and analgesic nephropathy.

Secondary
Obstructive uropathy.

Vascular disorders

Renal artery stenosis
Due to atherosclerosis, fibromuscular dysplasia, thrombosis and Takayasu's syndrome.

Vasculitis
Due to polyarteritis, Wegener's granulomatosis, haemolytic uraemic syndrome, and progressive systemic sclerosis.

Pregnancy associated
Pre-eclamptic toxaemia and post-partum acute renal failure.

Metabolic disorders

Including diabetes mellitus, amyloidosis, multiple myeloma, calculus disease, and gout.

Developmental disorders

Including polycystic disease and renal dysplasia.

Renin-producing tumours

These are very rare causes of hypertension, and are not discussed further.

End-stage renal disease

This results from any of the above disease processes.

70 Normal renal cortex consisting of the glomerulus, surrounded predominantly by proximal tubules and distal tubules at the glomerular hilum (between 4 and 5 o'clock to the glomerulus) (H & E × 100).

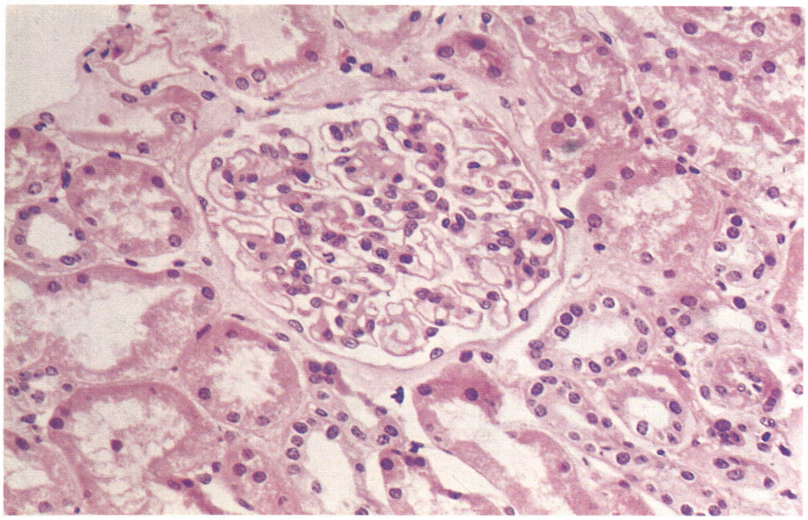

70

71 Normal renal glomerulus consisting of a capillary tuft within Bowman's capsule. Capillary walls are thin, lumina widely patent, and supporting mesangium scanty (PAS × 400).

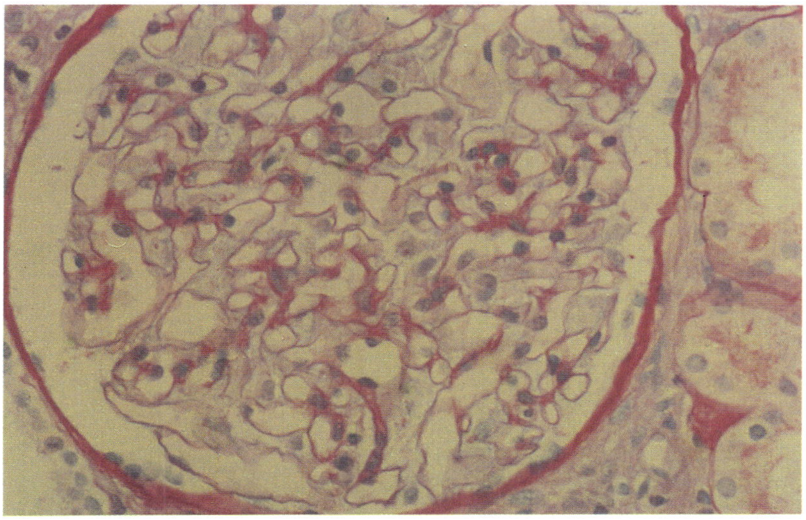

71

Acute proliferative post-streptococcal glomerulonephritis

72

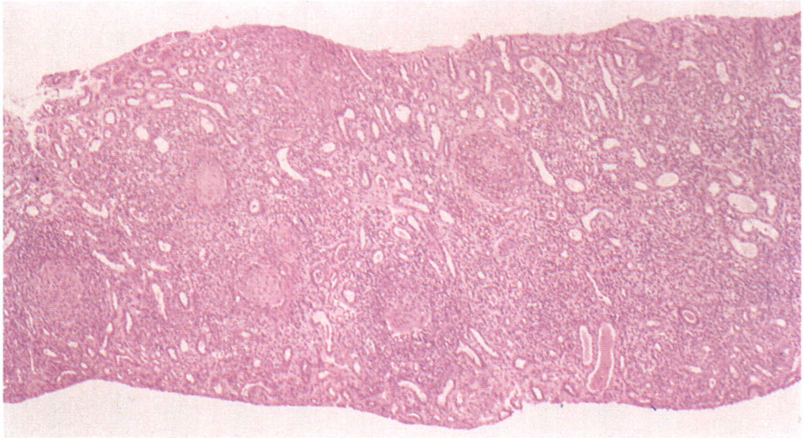

72 Low power view of a biopsy from a patient with acute post-streptococcal glomerulonephritis. All the glomeruli are diffusely abnormal (H & E × 40).

73

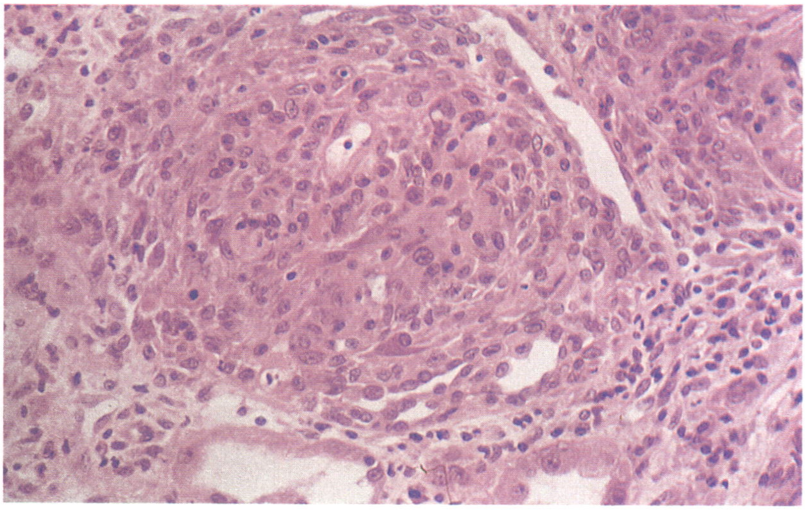

73 High power view of a glomerulus which is enlarged, hypercellular, and has occlusion of capillary lumina (H & E × 400).

74

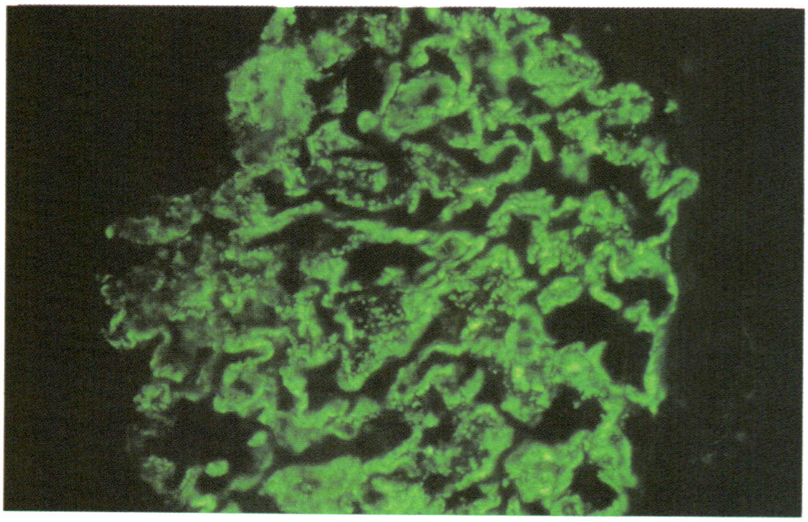

74 Diffuse, granular deposits of immune complexes on glomerular capillary walls; positive staining for IgG. (Immunofluorescent stain × 400).

75

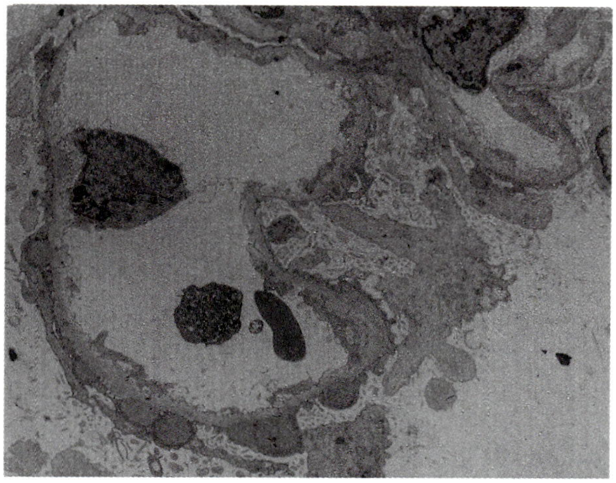

75 Electron micrograph of a single glomerular capillary loop showing large immune complex deposits on the outer aspect of the wall (× 2800).

76

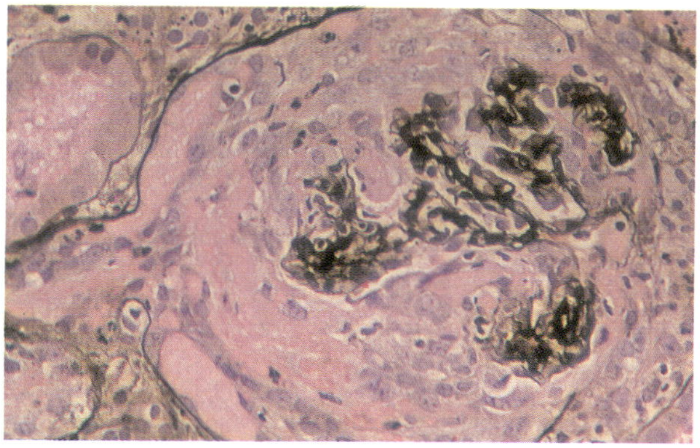

76 Destruction and necrosis of capillary walls with leakage of fibrin into Bowman's space, which evokes proliferation of cells to form crescents. Capillary walls are stained black with silver stain (× 400)

77

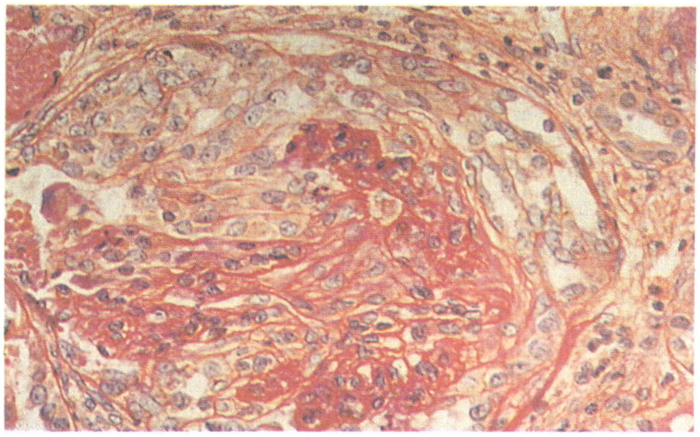

77 Glomerulus with changes similar to **75** (PAS × 400).

78

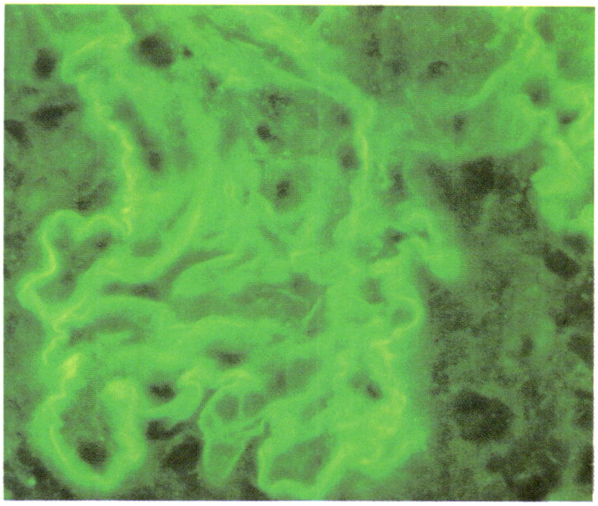

78 Diffuse linear immunofluorescent staining of glomerular capillary walls for IgG, diagnostic of anti-GBM nephritis (× 400).

Lupus Nephritis

79

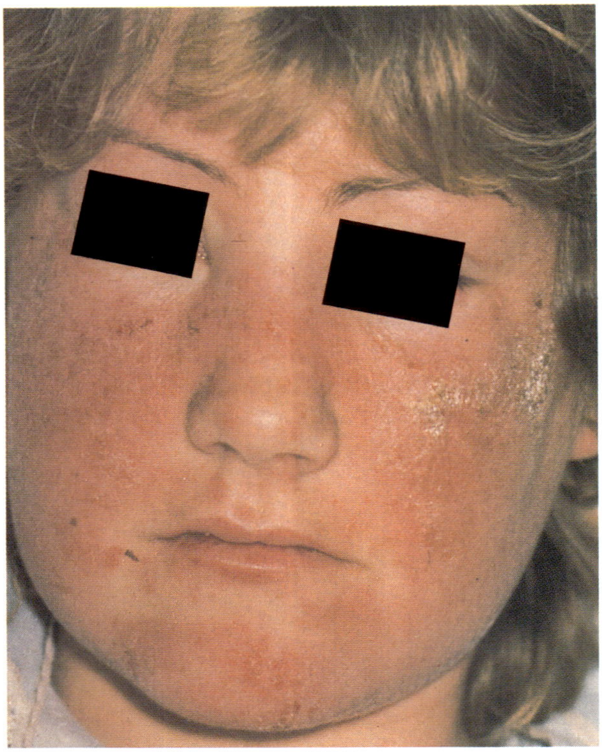

80

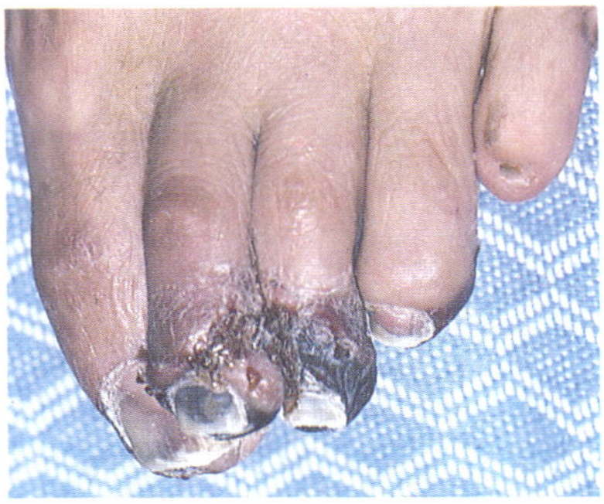

80 Small vessel disease may lead to digital gangrene in SLE.

79 Clinical photograph of young female with systemic lupus erythematosus (SLE) showing a typical butterfly rash.

81

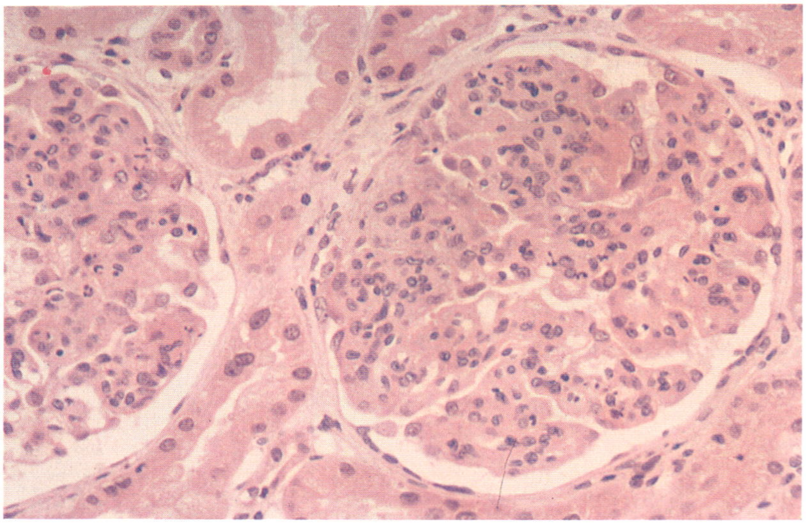

81 Diffusely hypercellular and enlarged glomeruli consistent with diffuse proliferative lupus nephritis (H & E × 200).

82 Hypercellular glomerulus with some capillary walls markedly thickened and rigid wire loop abnormality (PAS × 400).

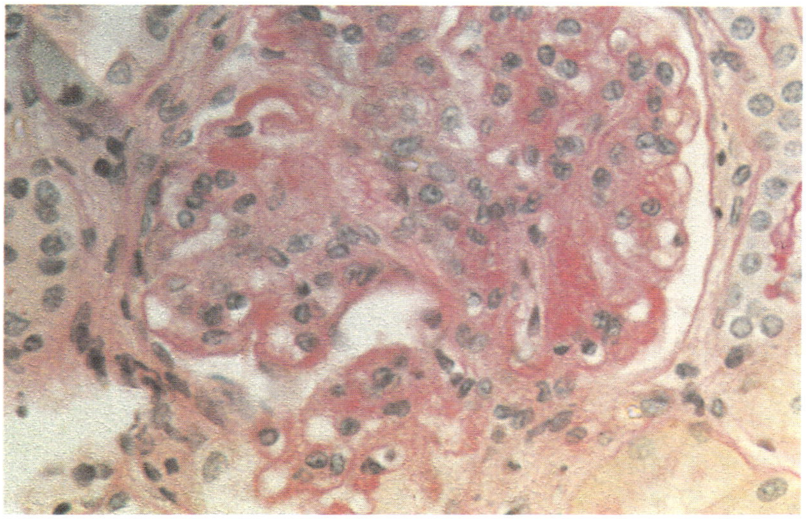

82

83

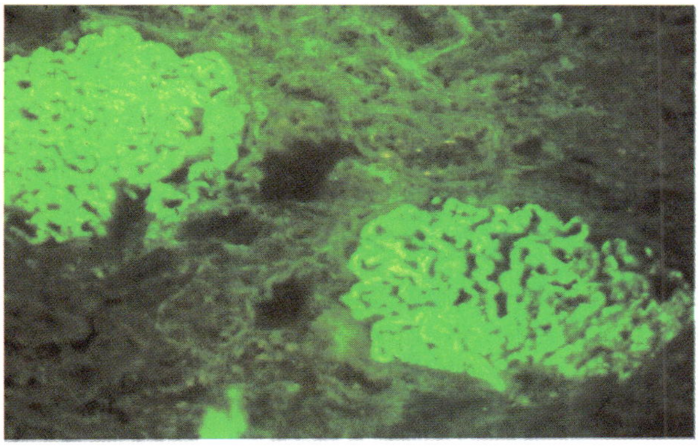

83 Diffuse brilliant granular staining of capillary walls for IgG, typical of an immune complex glomerulonephritis (× 200).

84

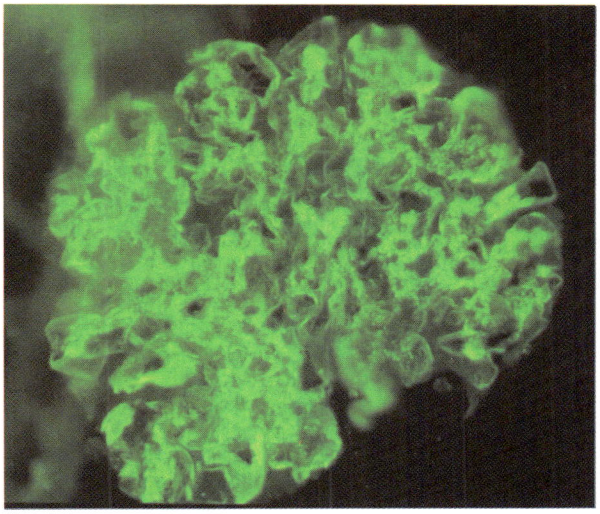

84 Staining for C_3 in a case similar to **83** (× 400).

85

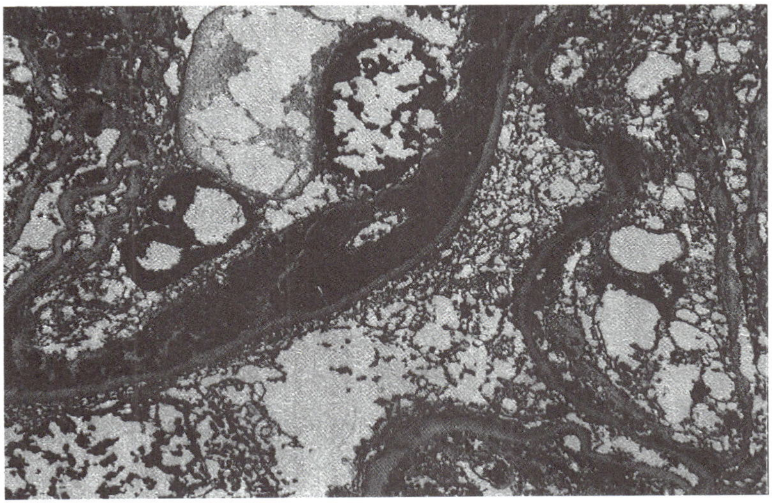

85 Electron micrograph showing large, ribbon-like deposition of immune complexes along the inner endothelial aspect of capillary walls, equivalent to the wire loop lesions seen with light microscopy (× 4800).

86

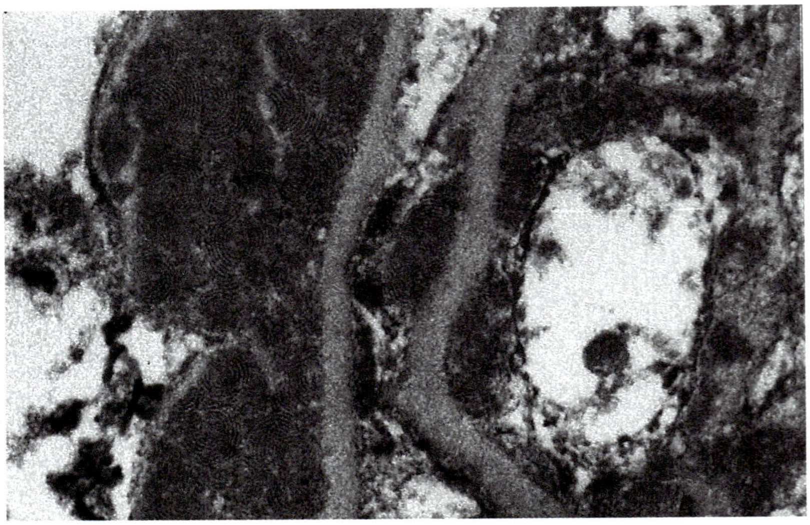

86 Very large deposits with crystalline structure (thumb print appearances) on both outer (epithelial) and inner (endothelial) aspect of capillary walls. Such deposits are diagnostic of lupus nephritis (× 8600).

87

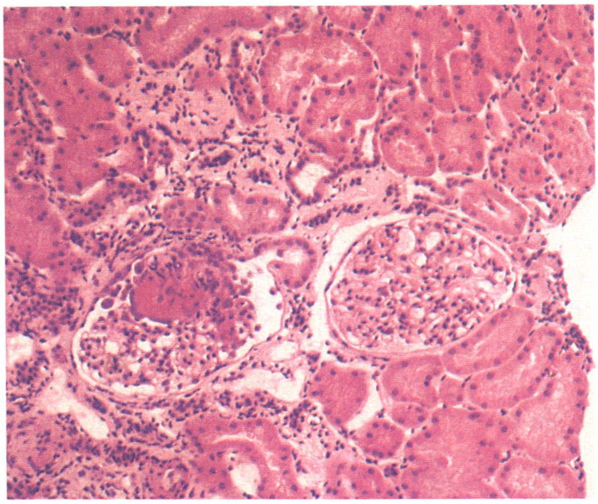

87 Two glomeruli, one normal and the other showing focal proliferative and necrotizing glomerulonephritis, in which there is necrosis and destruction of capillary loops within a segment of the glomerulus together with foci of cellular proliferation. This abnormality can be seen in a number of conditions, including lupus nephritis, polyarteritis nodosa, Wegener's granulomatosis and Henoch–Schönlein syndrome (H & E × 400).

88

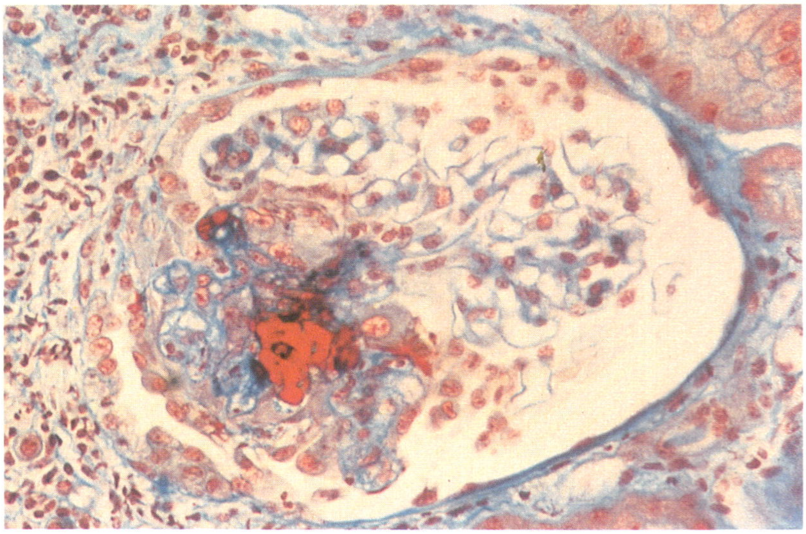

88 Glomerulus similar to **87**, stained with MSB, which stains fibrin red (× 400).

Chronic end-stage glomerulonephritis

89

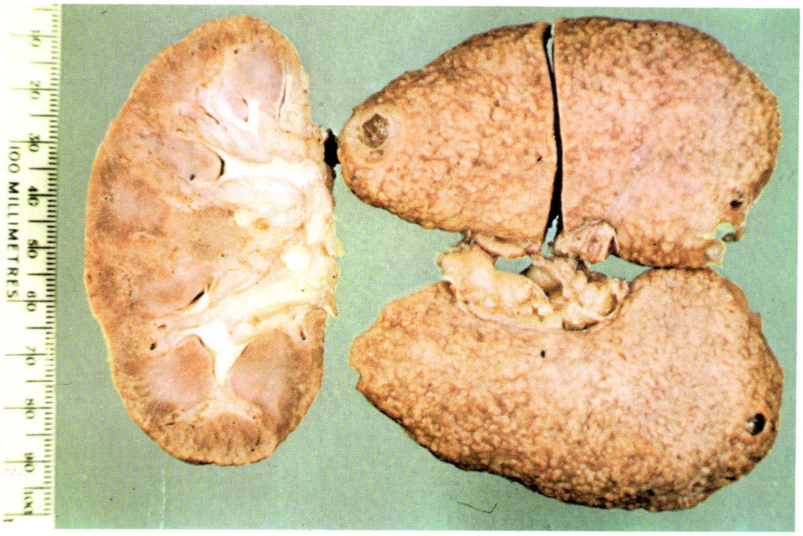

90

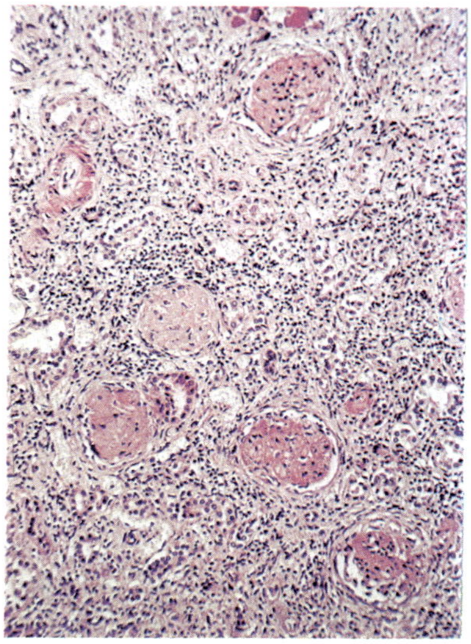

89 The kidneys are of a similar size, small, 6–7 cm length (normally 12 cm), and have a marked decrease in renal parenchyma with an increase in pelvic adipose tissue. The surface is diffusely granular.

90 Low power view of chronic end-stage glomerulonephritis. There is marked sclerosis of glomeruli, tubular atrophy, non-specific interstitial inflammation, and thickening of arterial walls (PAS × 40).

91

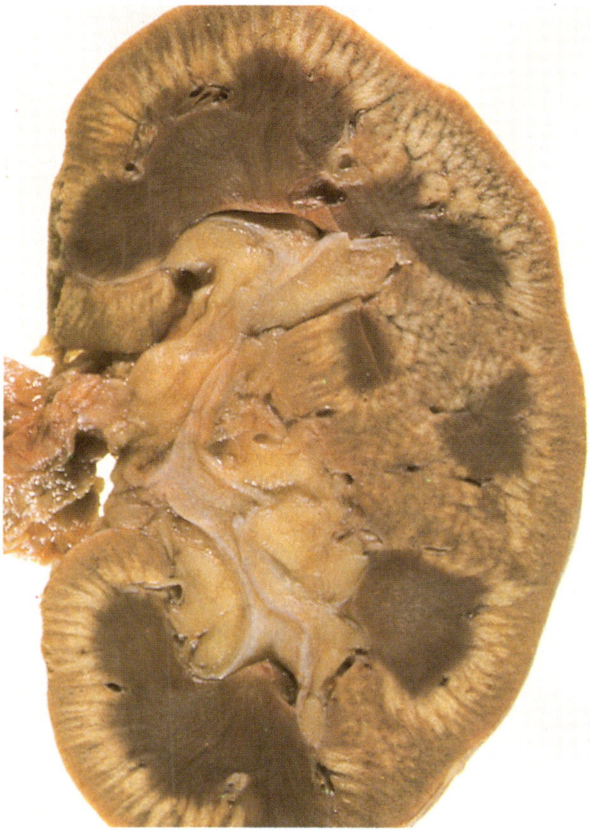

91 Long-standing membranous glomerulonephritis in which a patient had nephrotic syndrome but without established renal failure. The kidney is slightly enlarged with a yellow, streaky, widened cortex. The yellow colour is due to the filtration of lipoproteins, which are deposited in the tubular epithelium.

92 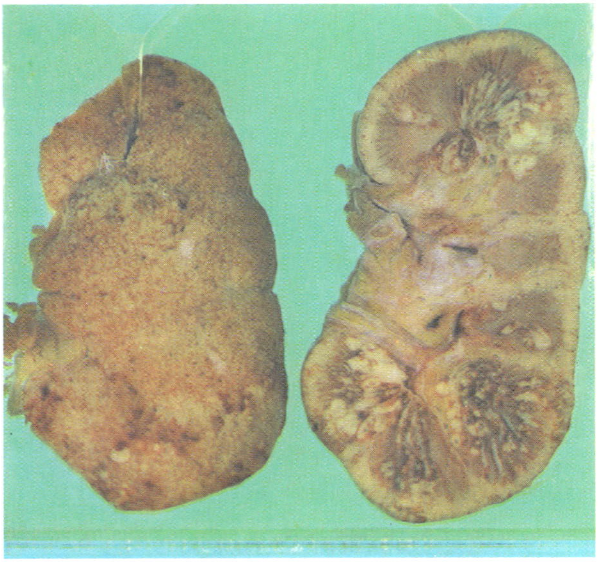

92 Macroscopic section in acute pyelonephritis (PN). Multiple streaks of yellow pus in the medulla of upper and lower poles are intermingled with more obvious abscesses. The streaks are indicative of ascending infection with intrarenal reflux of white cell casts.

93 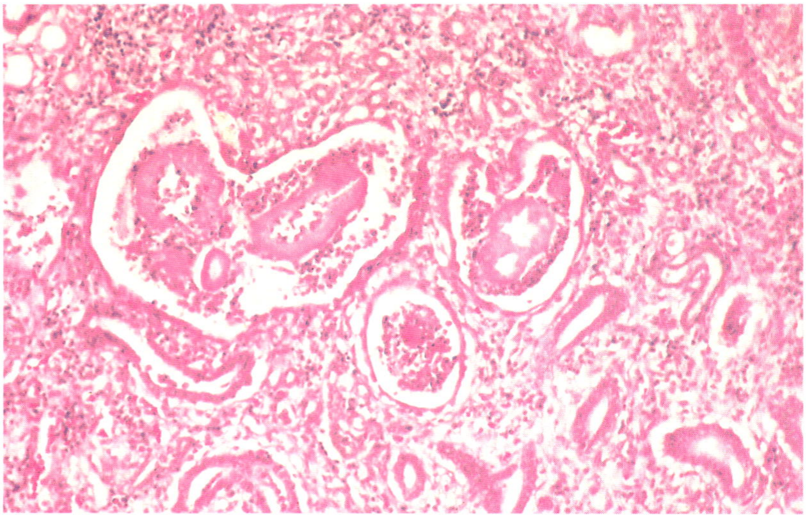

93 Acute PN histology. Tubular lumina contain white cell casts and necrotic epithelial debris and the interstitium is heavily infiltrated by neutrophils and some lymphocytes (H & E × 100).

94 Chronic reflux nephropathy. Both kidneys are reduced in size but unequal. Calyces at the poles are distorted (particularly in the smaller kidney) with scarring of the overlying parenchyma. The parenchymal damage is due to repeated intrarenal reflux of urine. The reflux is due either to a primary structural abnormality of the calyces, or urinary outflow obstruction, which increases intrapelvic pressure.

94

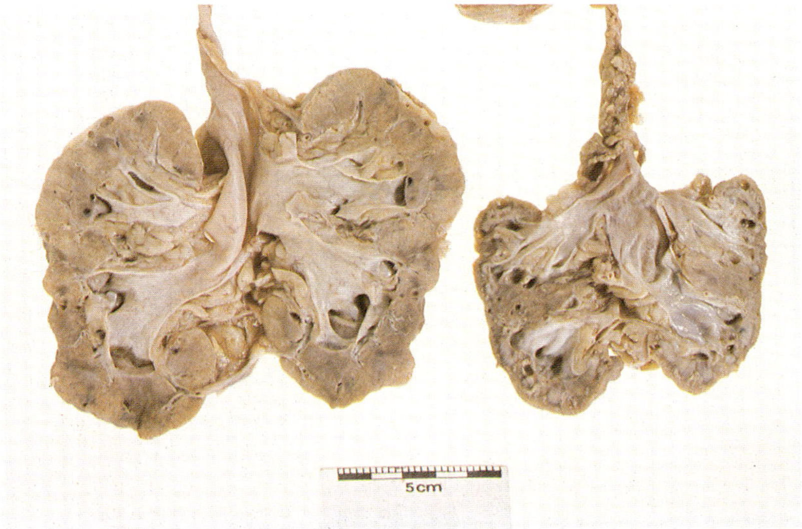

95 Low power view of radiating parenchymal scarring caused by intrarenal reflux (very early changes) (H & E × 100).

95

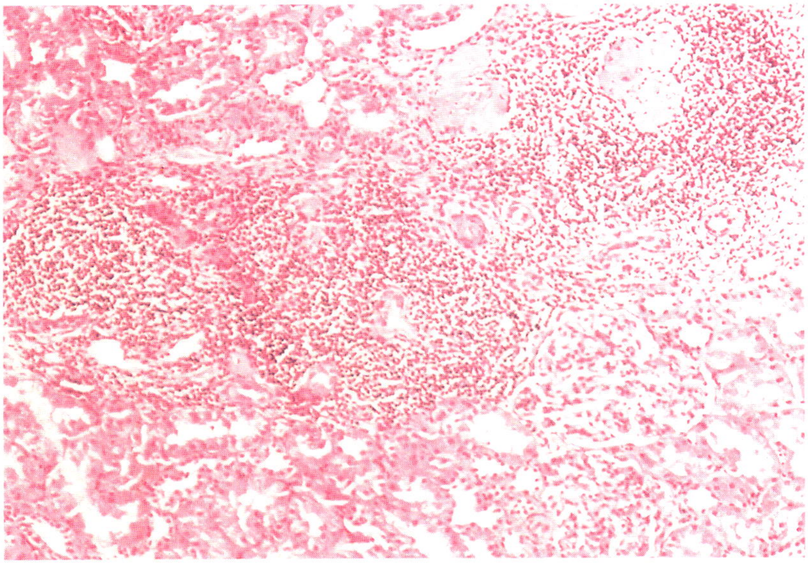

96 Intravenous urogram showing a normal left nephrogram and a small right kidney due to chronic reflux nephropathy.

96

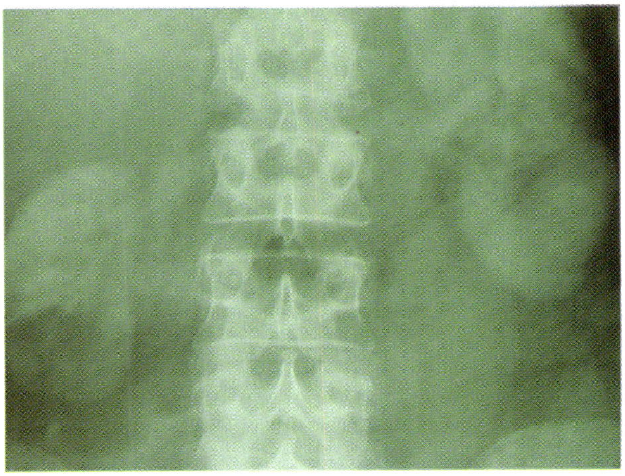

97

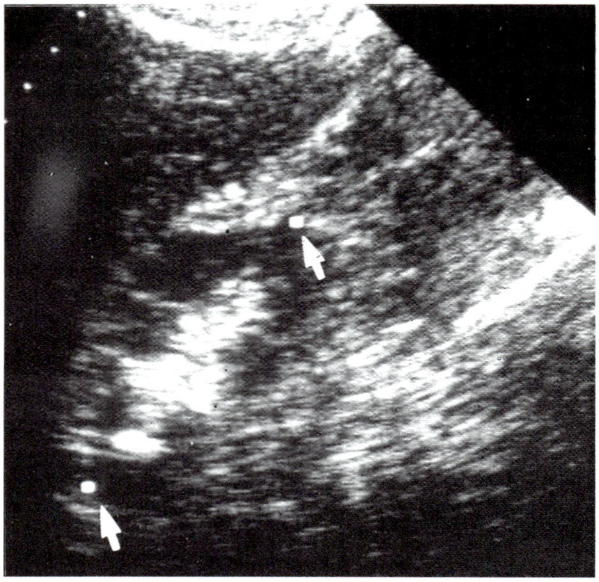

97 Renal size may be readily measured by ultrasound. The white dots (arrows) situated at the upper and lower poles are 7.5 cm apart, representing a kidney shrunken by reflux nephropathy.

98

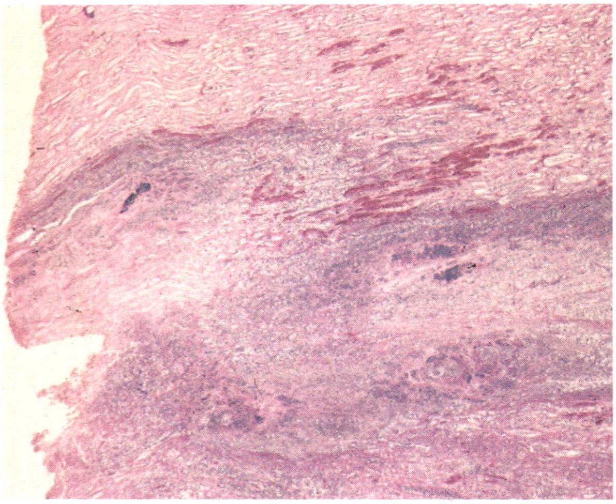

98 Acute papillary necrosis secondary to analgesic toxicity. The border zone at the edge of necrotic papilla is hypercellular, with intense infiltration of neutrophils (H & E × 40).

99

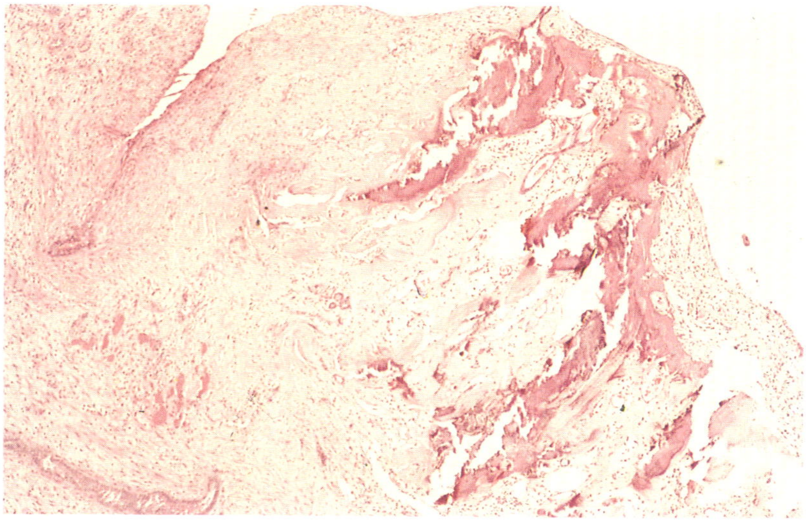

99 Healed papillary necrosis showing distorted and mummified necrotic papilla with dystrophic bone formation (H & E × 100).

100 Intravenous urogram in analgesic nephropathy, in this case due to phenacetin, showing distorted clubbed calyces in the right kidney.

100

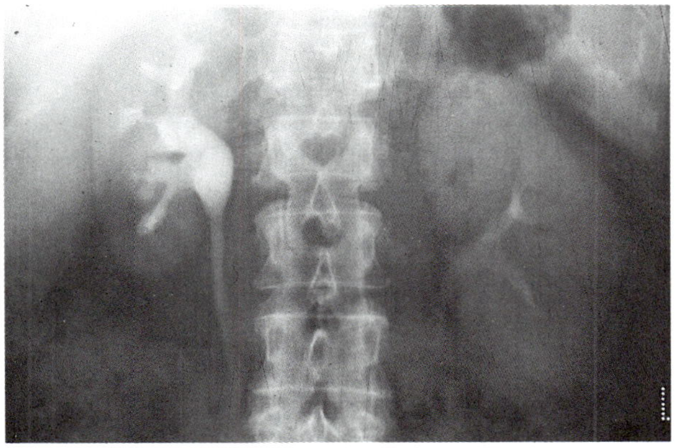

101

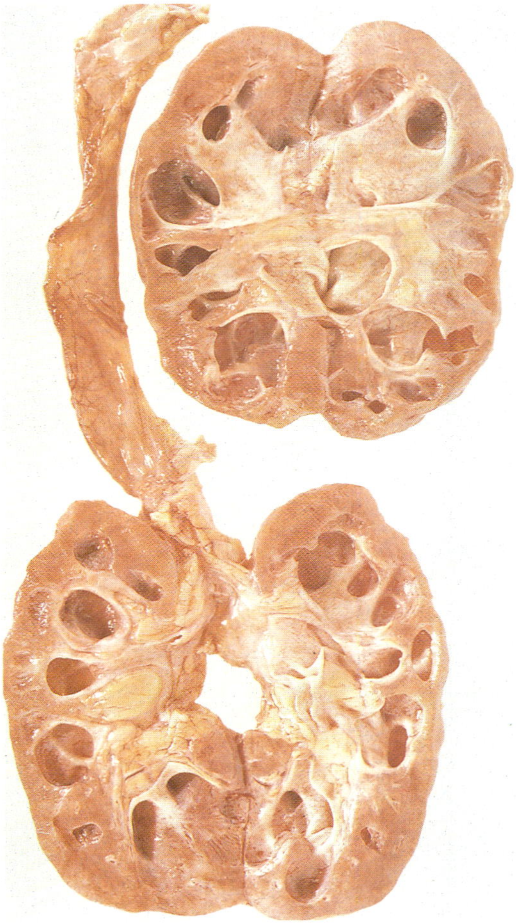

101 Hydronephrosis: there is a dilated pelvicalyceal system, and the cortex and medulla are markedly thinned.

102

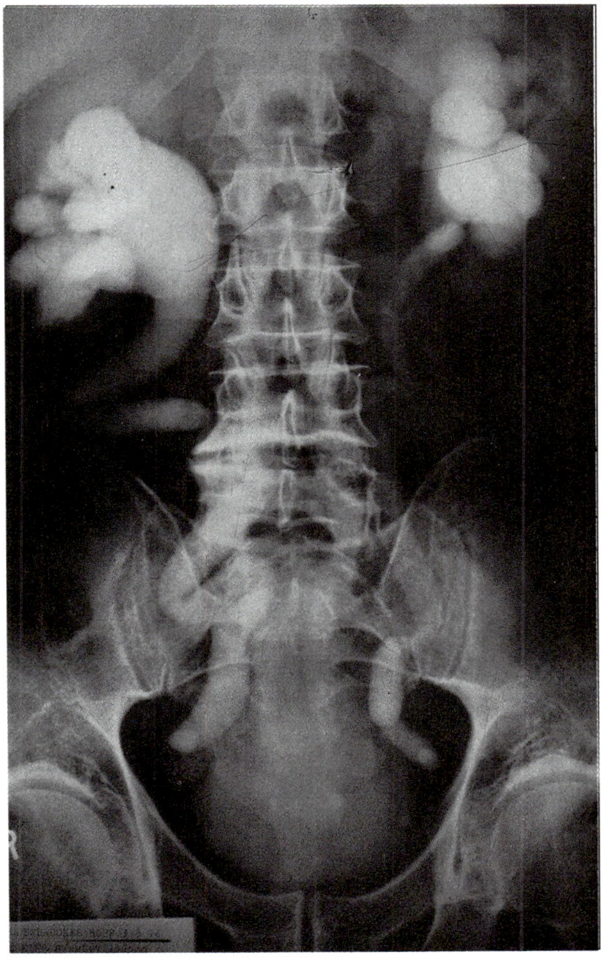

102 Intravenous urogram in a patient with bladder neck obstruction due to prostatic enlargement. There is bilateral hydronephrosis.

103

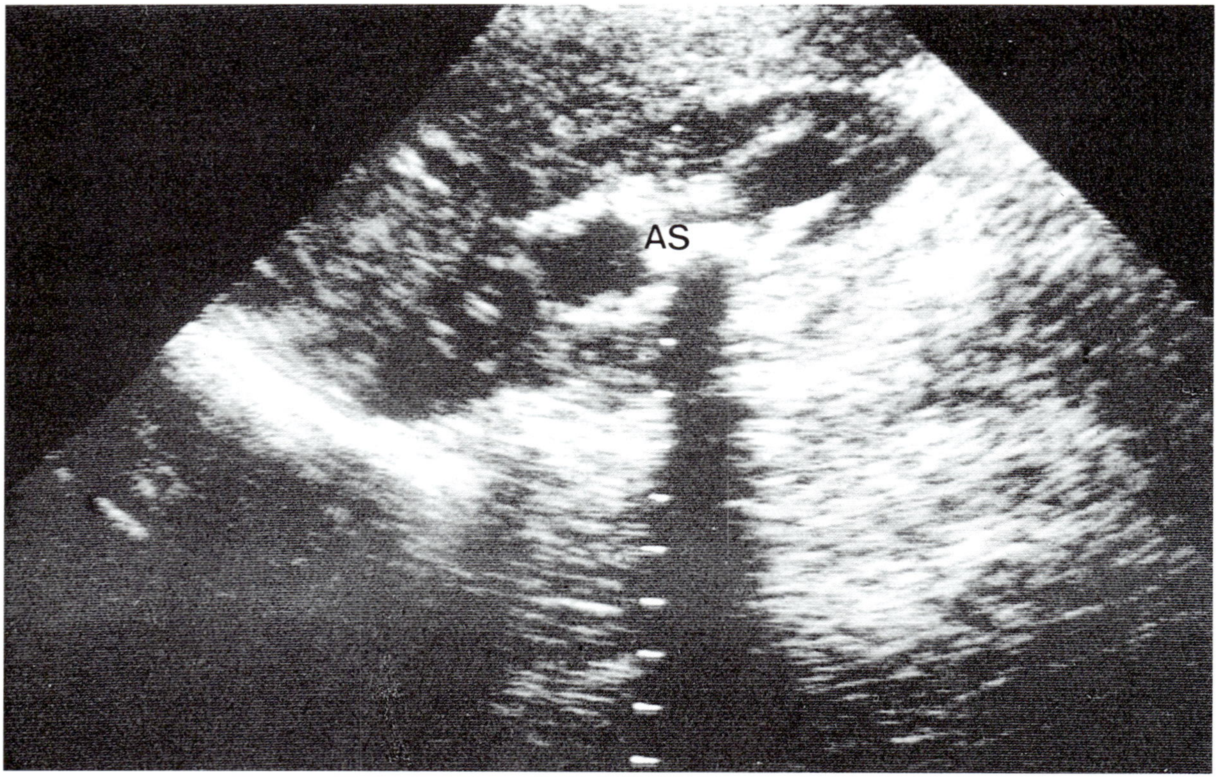

103 Ultrasound image in hydronephrosis. The calyces are dilated (DC) and an acoustic shadow (AS) corresponds to a renal calculus.

104

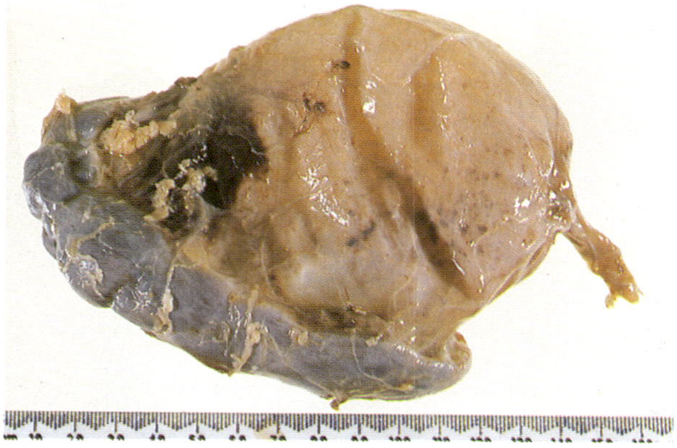

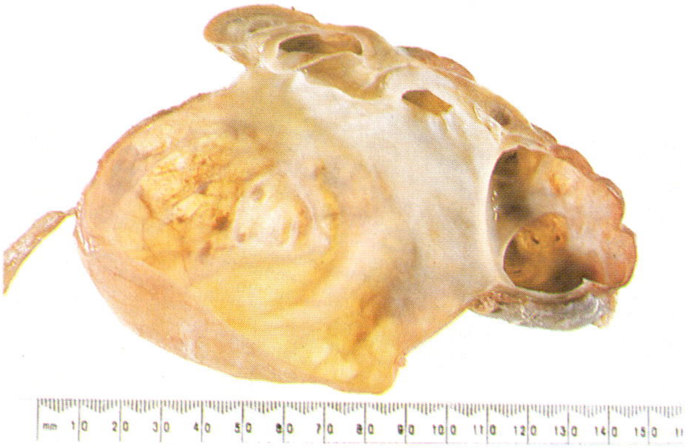

104 , 105 Macroscopic appearance of a severe, long-standing pelvi-ureteric junction obstruction. Note the normal calibre ureter with abrupt massive dilatation of the pelvis and calyces with total destruction of renal parenchyma.

106 Intravenous urogram in a pelvi-ureteric junction obstruction with dilatation above the obstruction and a normal distal ureter.

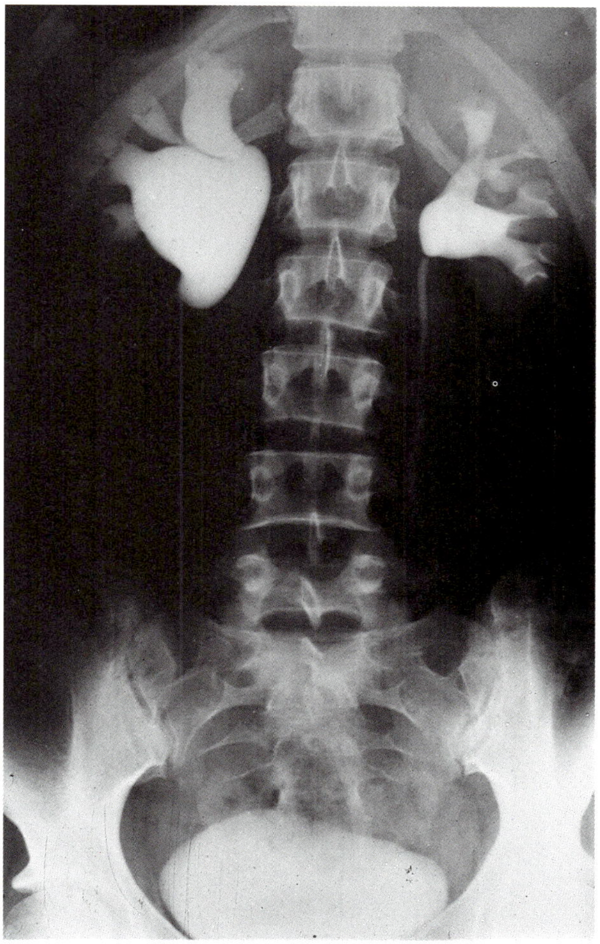

106

Vasculitis

107 Polyarteritis nodosa (PAN) may have a wide variety of clinical manifestations. Shown here is a vasculitic skin rash.

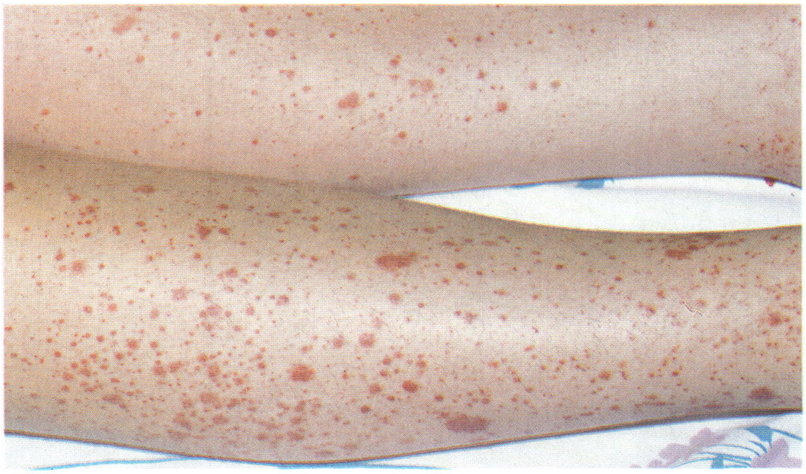

107

108

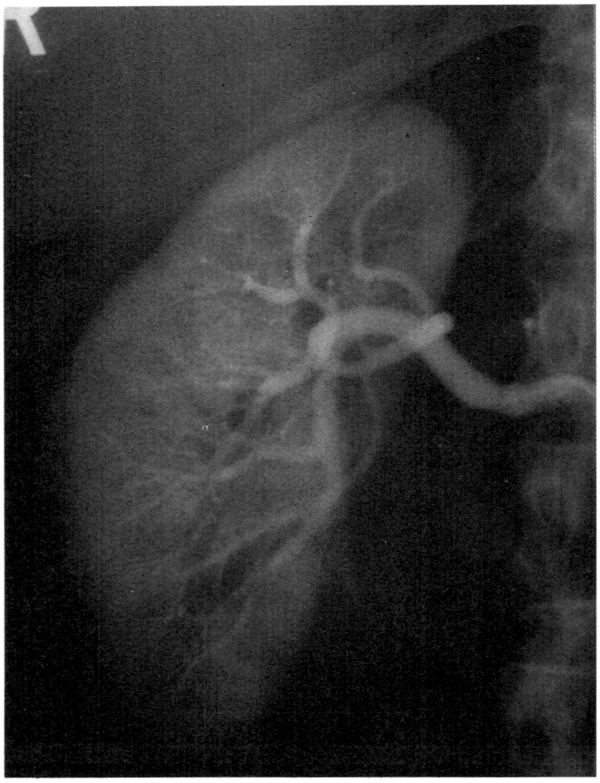

109

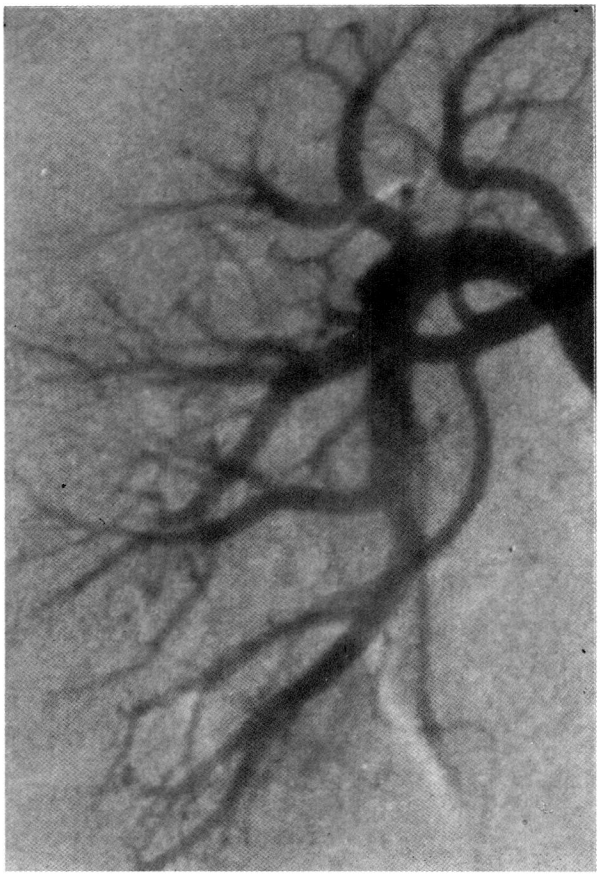

110

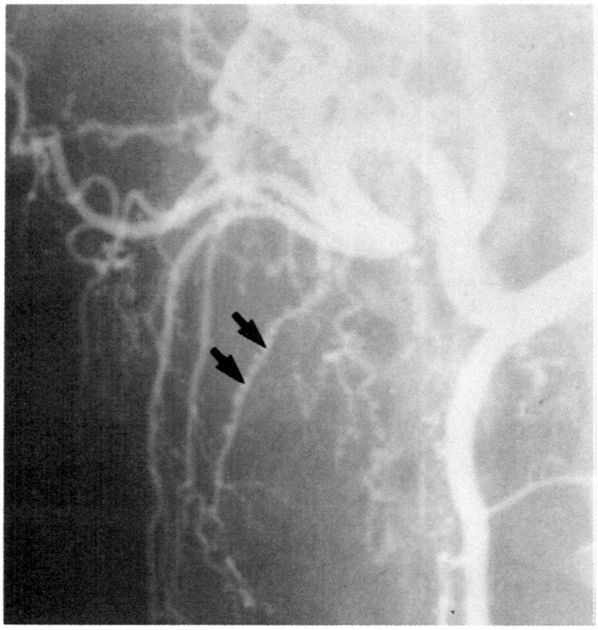

108–110 The small arterial aneurysms typical of this condition may be demonstrated by angiography, with a beaded arterial appearance in both kidneys (**108, 109**), better shown in the liver (**110**).

111

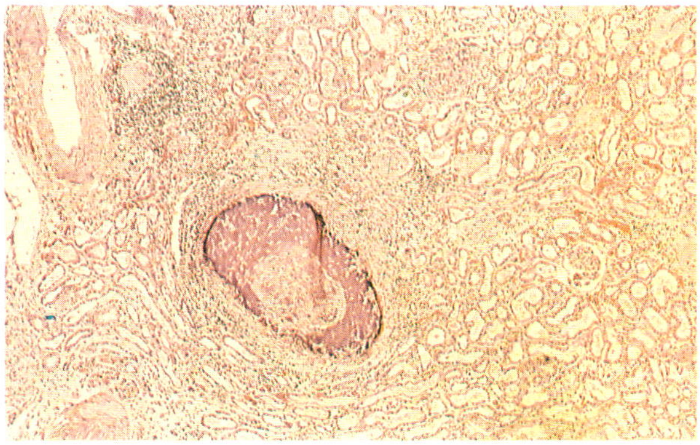

112

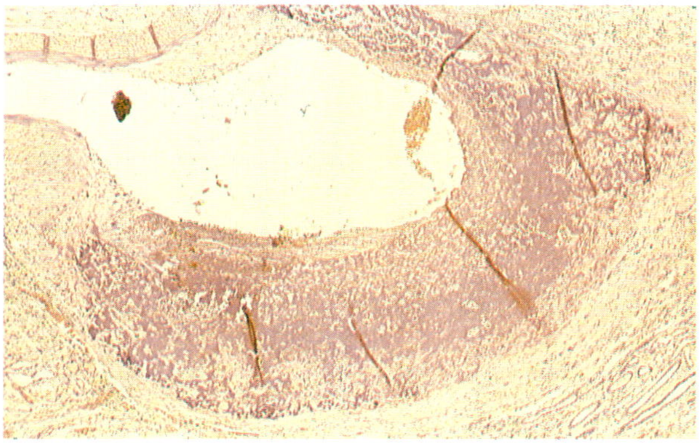

111 Low power section of renal polyarteritis. There is circumferential, fibrinoid necrosis of the wall of an interlobar artery with surrounding inflammation. The lumen is occluded by thrombus (H & E × 40).

112 Higher power view of fibrinoid necrosis of an artery in PAN. Most of the wall is structureless, intensely eosinophilic (fibrinous), and shows early aneurysmal dilatation (H & E × 200).

113

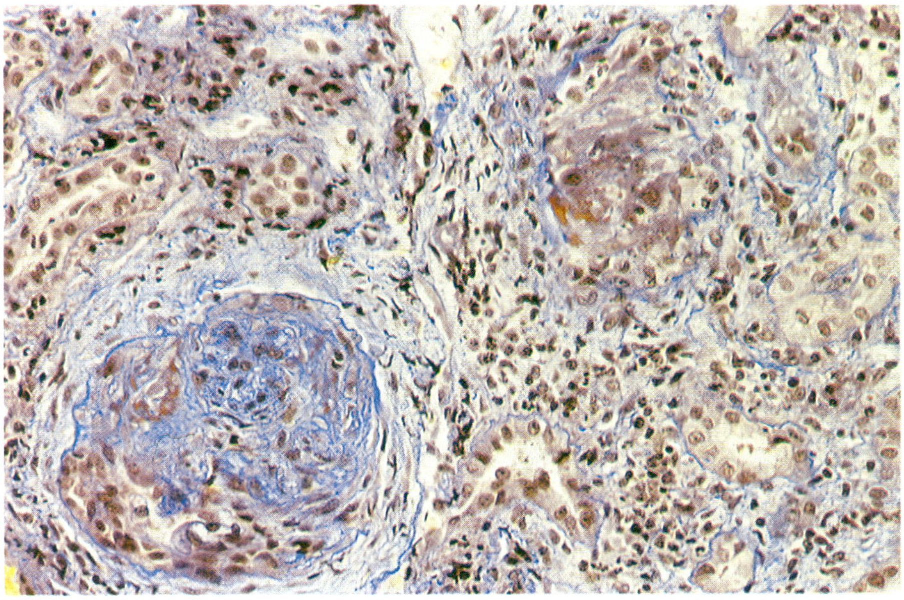

113 Global necrosis of glomerulus in PAN (MSB × 200).

114

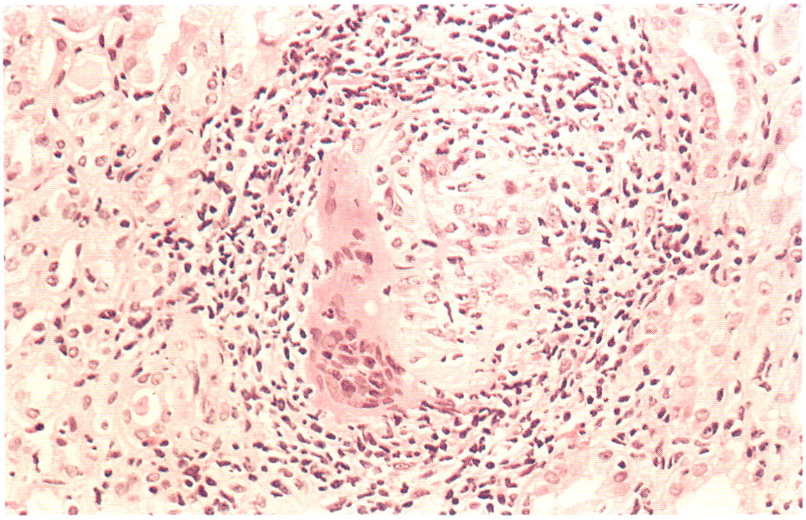

114 Unrecognizable, necrotic glomerulus in PAN replaced by a mass of inflammatory cells, including multinucleate giant cells (H & E × 400).

115

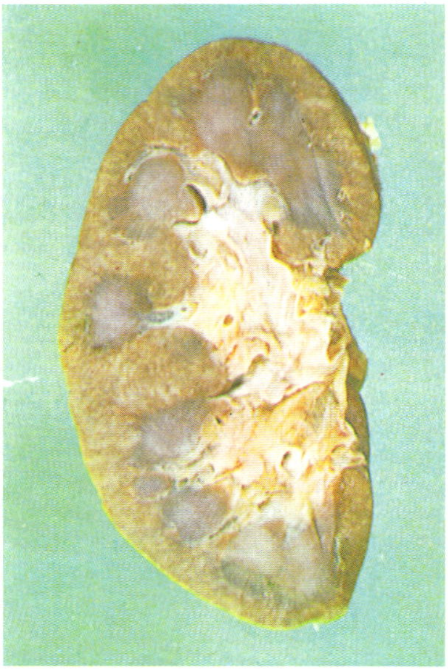

115 Hemisection of the kidney in progressive systolic sclerosis (PSS) showing normal renal size but a diffusely mottled cortex containing several minute infarcts.

116

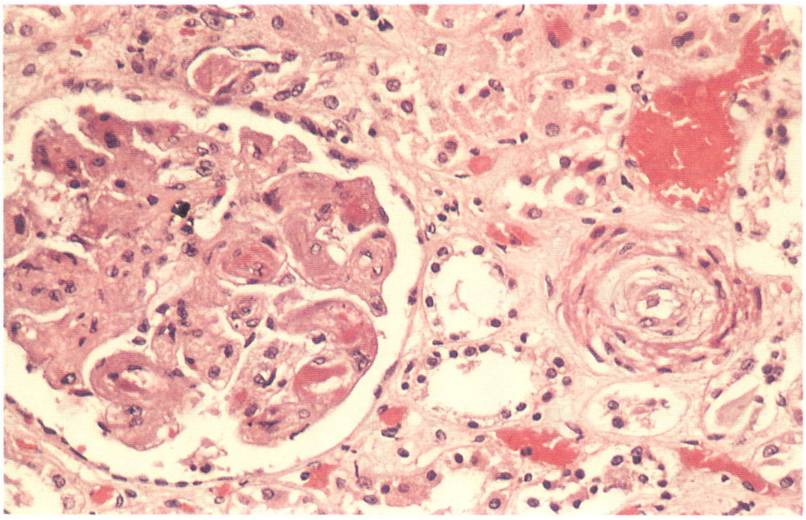

116 Kidney in PSS showing a severely abnormal arteriole with luminal narrowing secondary to the mucoid, and concentric myointimal thickening of the wall. The glomerulus shows sludging of red cells and fibrin within capillary loops (H & E × 200).

117

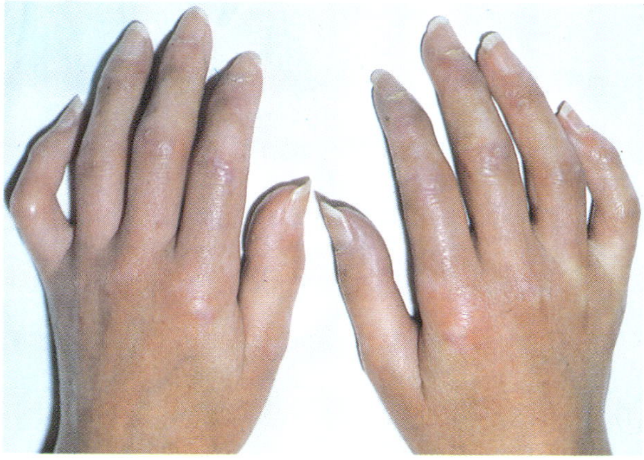

117 The hand in systemic sclerosis shows thickening and tightening of the skin, particularly around the finger.

118

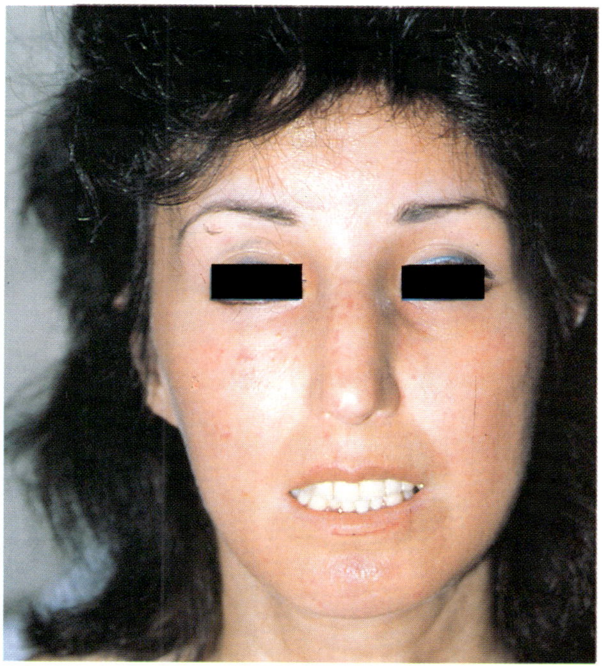

118 The facial appearance in systemic sclerosis includes stretched skin, especially around the mouth.

119

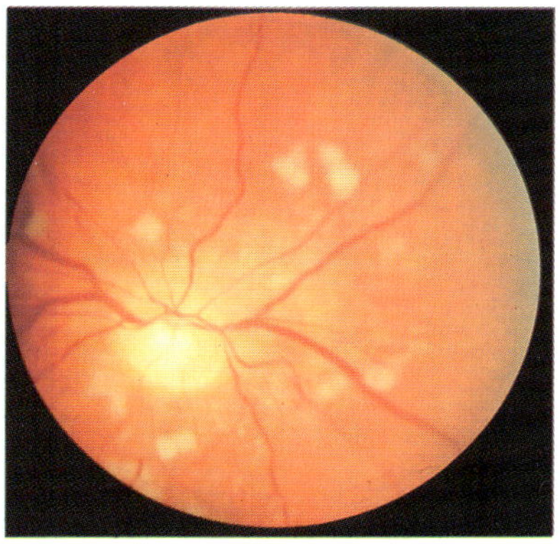

119 In scleroderma, there may be widespread soft exudates in the retina.

Metabolic disorders

120

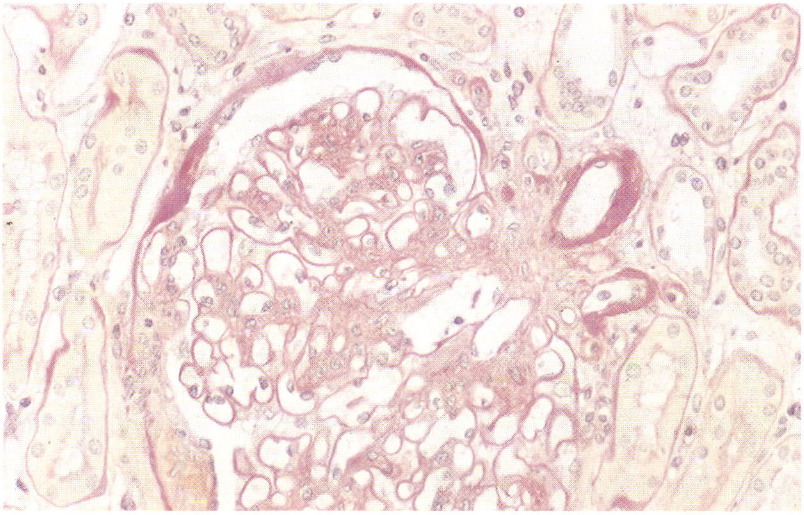

120 Early diabetic glomerulosclerosis with a moderate mesangial matrical increase and sclerosis of the afferent and efferent arterioles at the hilum (PAS × 200).

121

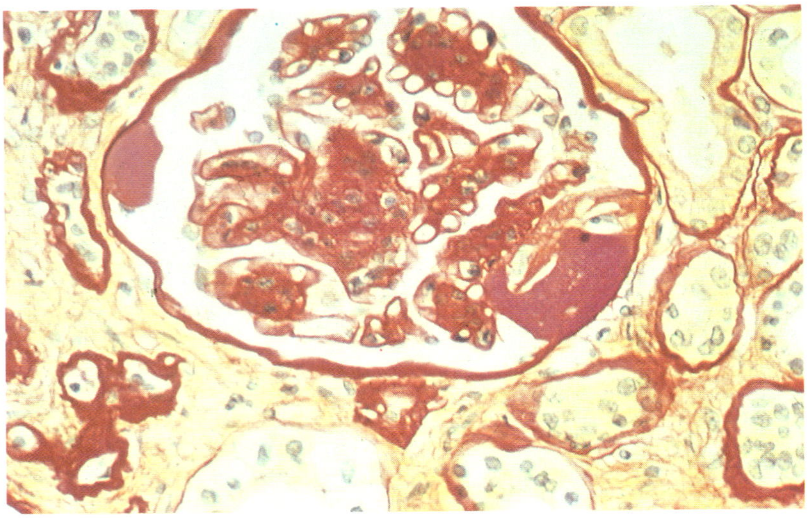

121 More advanced diabetic glomerulosclerosis with a prominent diffuse mesangial matrical increase and nodular accentuation at 1 o'clock. At 4 and 9 o'clock there are nodular capsular drops, which are typical of diabetic glomerulosclerosis. Note the thickening of the tubular basement membrane with early atrophy (PAS × 400).

122

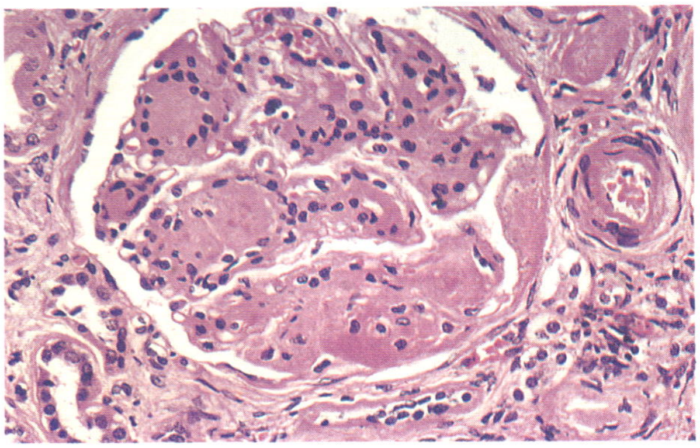

123

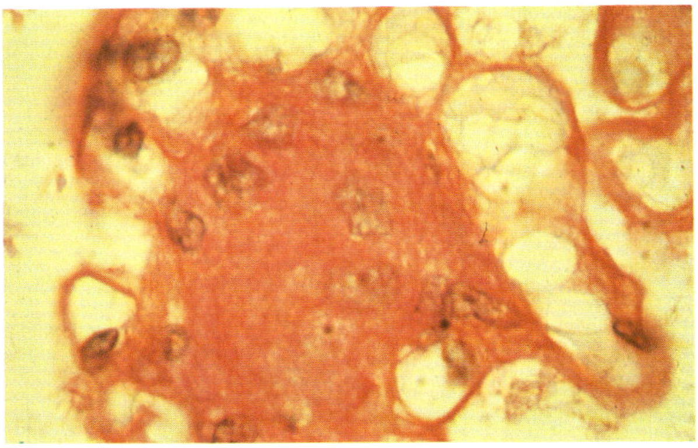

122 Nodular diabetic glomerulosclerosis (Kimmelstiel–Wilson lesion) with capsular drop and hilar arteriolar sclerosis (H & E × 400).

123 High power view of a single nodule illustrating the increase in mesangial matrix. The walls of the capillary loops are of normal thickness by light microscopy, and there is aneurysmal dilatation of the loop at 2–4 o'clock (PAS × 400).

124

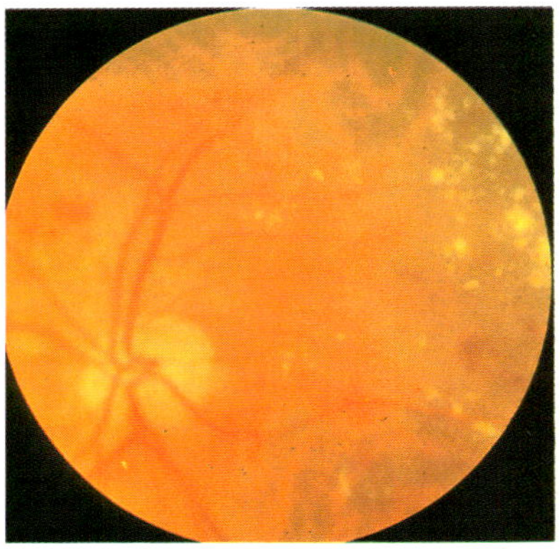

124, 125 Retinal photographs in diabetes mellitus showing cotton wool spots and micro aneurysms in background retinopathy (**124**). In the most severe forms of proliferative diabetic retinopathy, often associated with advanced renal disease, there are extensive areas of new vessel formation with large areas of haemorrhage. This patient has undergone photocoagulation (**125**).

125

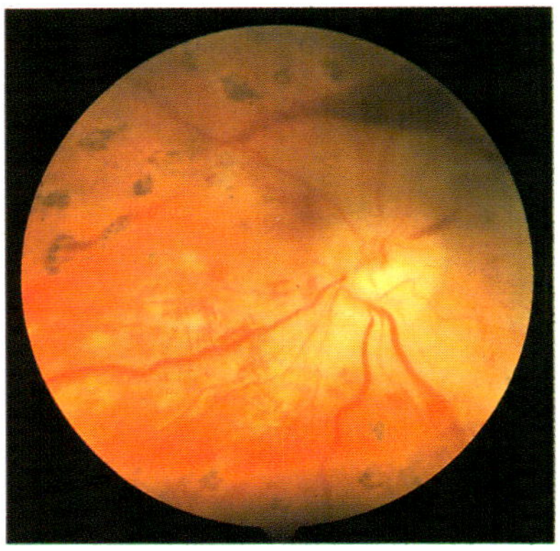

126

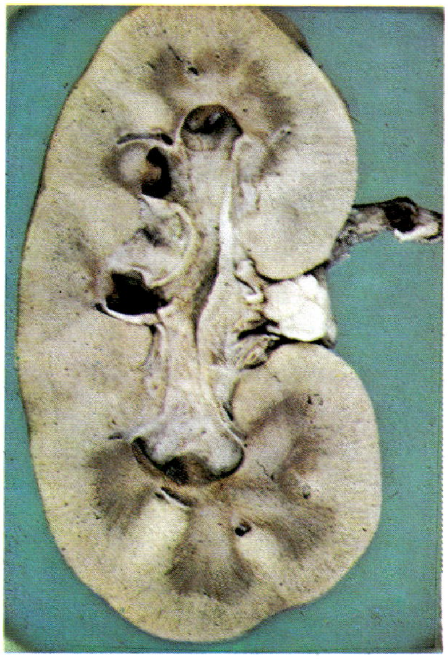

127

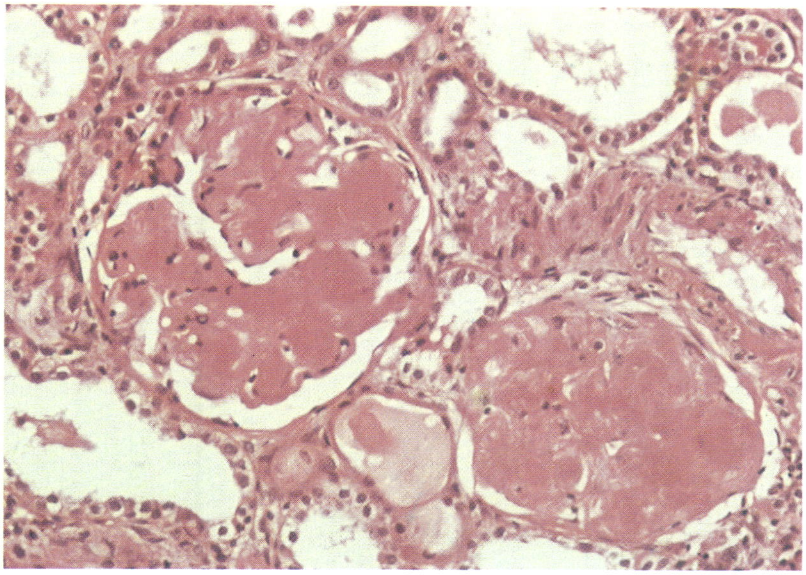

126 Macroscopic section of a hemisected kidney showing the characteristic wide pale cortex of amyloidosis.

127 Renal amyloid showing two acellular eosinophilic glomeruli without recognizable capillary loops. The eosinophilic nodular material represents amyloid (H & E × 200).

128 Congo red stain of renal amyloid viewed through polarizing lenses. Typical apple-green birefringence is indicative of amyloid in three glomeruli (Congo red × 100).

128

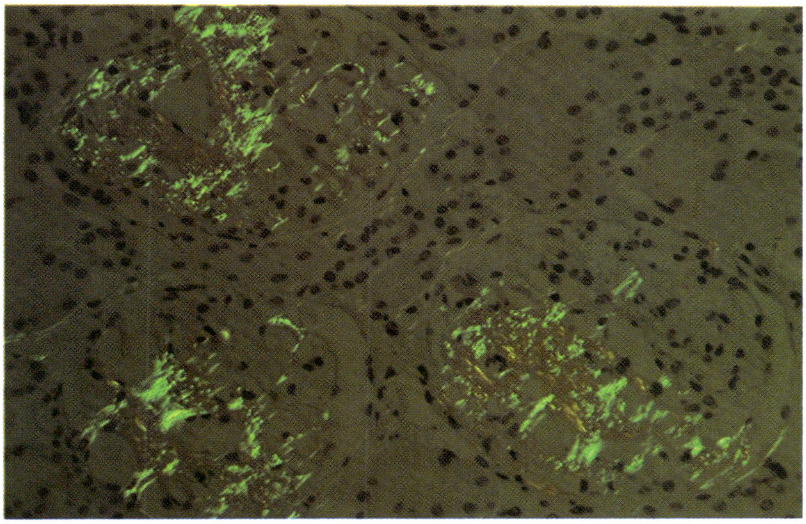

129

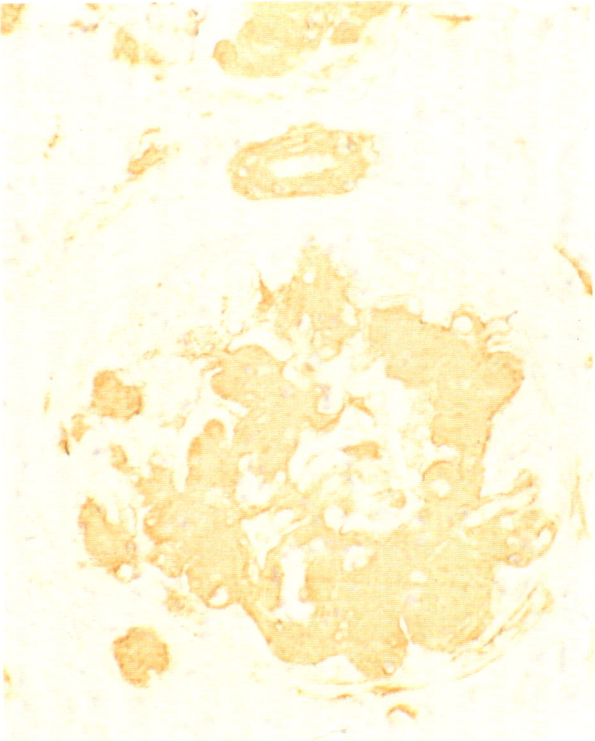

129 Immunoperoxidose stain of renal amyloid using monoclonal antibody against amyloid AA. Intense positive staining of glomerulus, arteriolar wall and some tubular basement membranes (× 100).

130

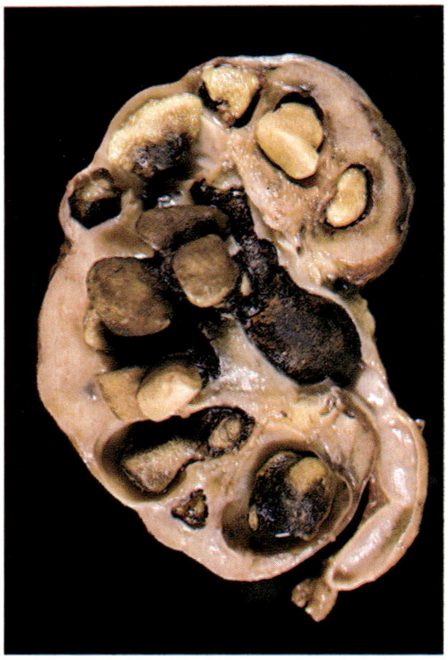

130 Macroscopic section of hydronephrosis and chronic pyelonephritis (reflux nephropathy) with stag-horn calculus. The dilated pelvis is filled with calculus and the cortex is paper thin in places.

13

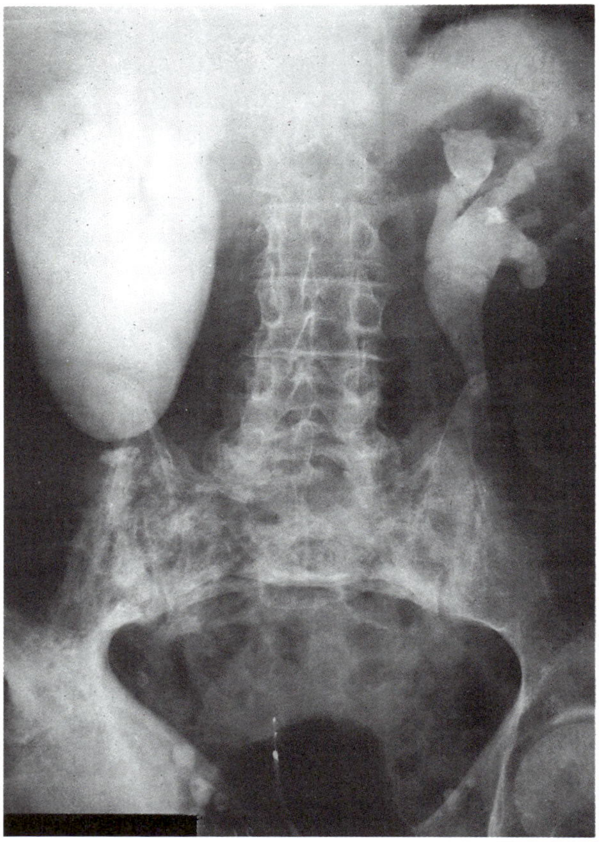

131 Huge stag-horn renal calculus in a patient with hypercalcaemia due to Paget's disease. Small calculi do not usually lead to renal hypertension.

132 Myeloma kidney showing typical casts of light chain proteins and cellular debris within tubular lumina. There is also a cellular reaction to these casts together with interstitial fibrosis and inflammation. The glomerulus is normal (H & E × 100).

132

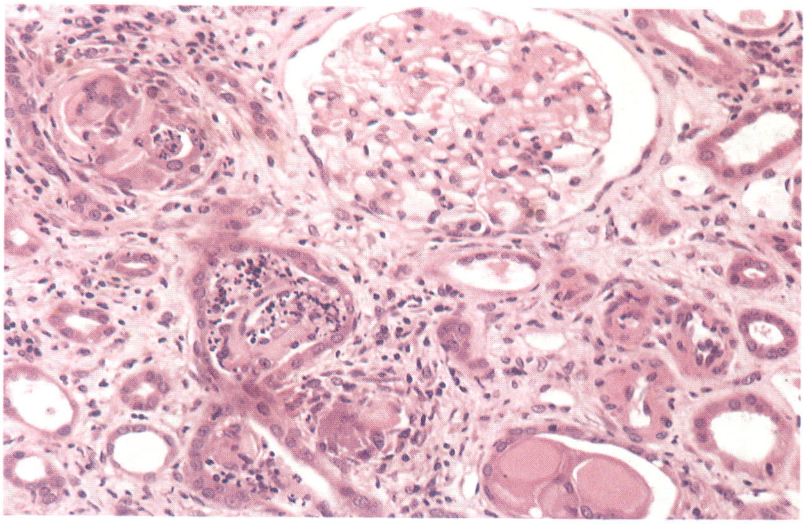

33

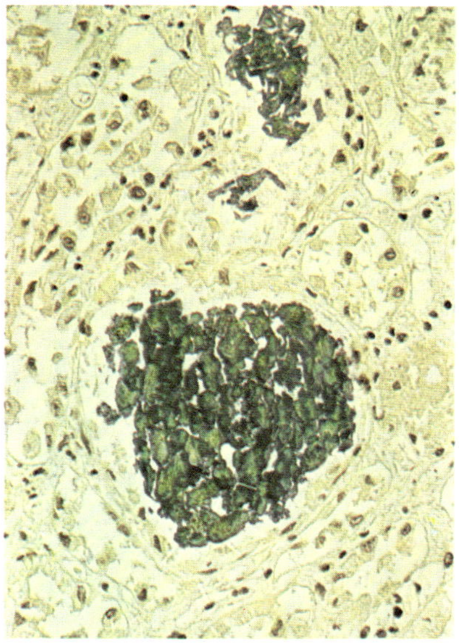

133–135 Renal involvement in gout may lead to hypertension. The histology of renal gout shows urate crystals giving a positive grey/green Schultz reaction (**133**). A gouty tophus is seen in the finger (**134**). In severe gout, there may be soft tissue swelling and bony erosions seen in the hand radiograph (**135**).

34

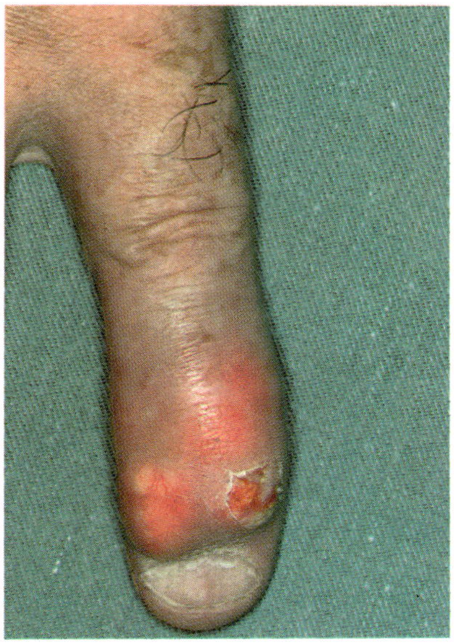

135

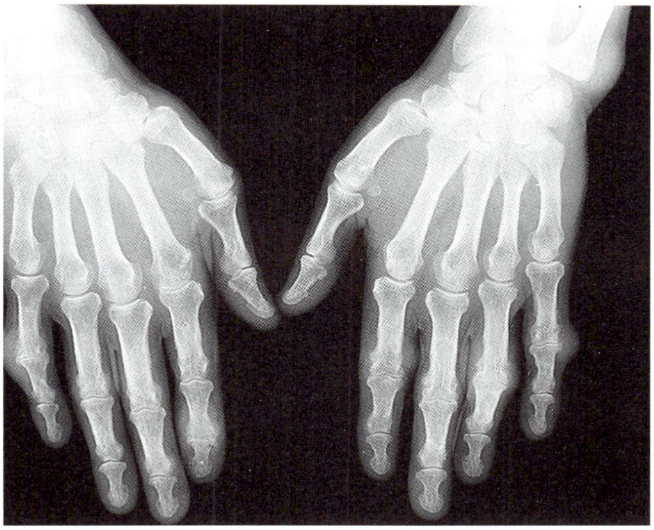

136

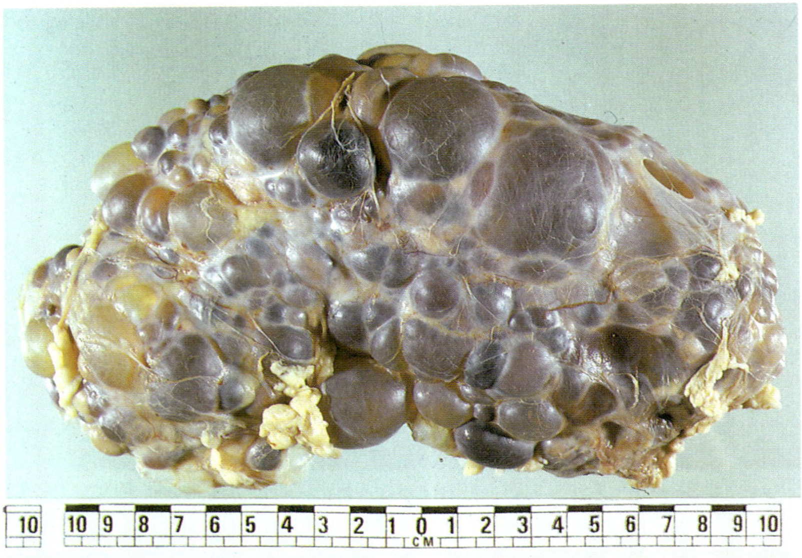

137

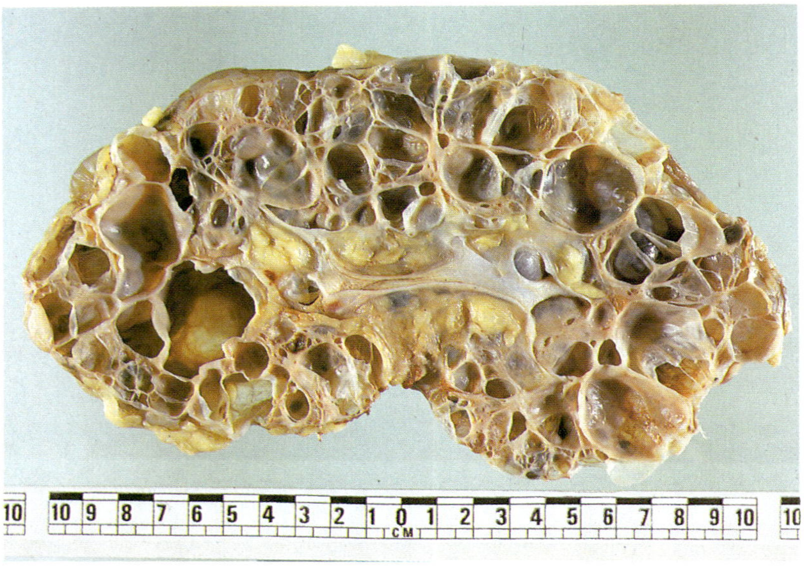

136, 137 External and cut surface of end-stage adult type polycystic kidney, which is enlarged (20–25 cm), and the renal parenchyma is entirely replaced by numerous thin-walled cysts. The two kidneys are invariably similar.

138

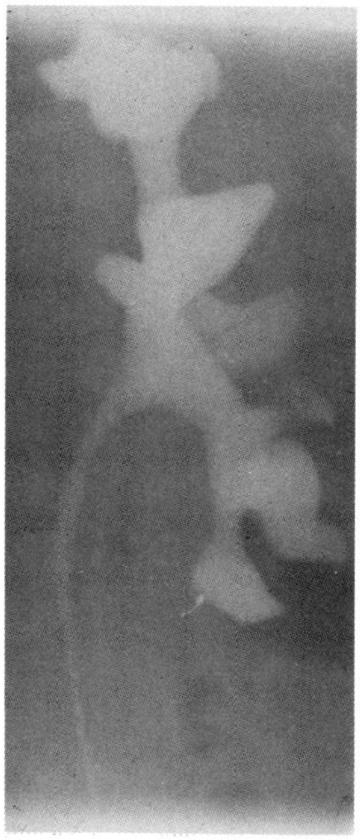

138 Retrograde urogram in polycystic disease with deformity of the pelvicalyceal system.

139

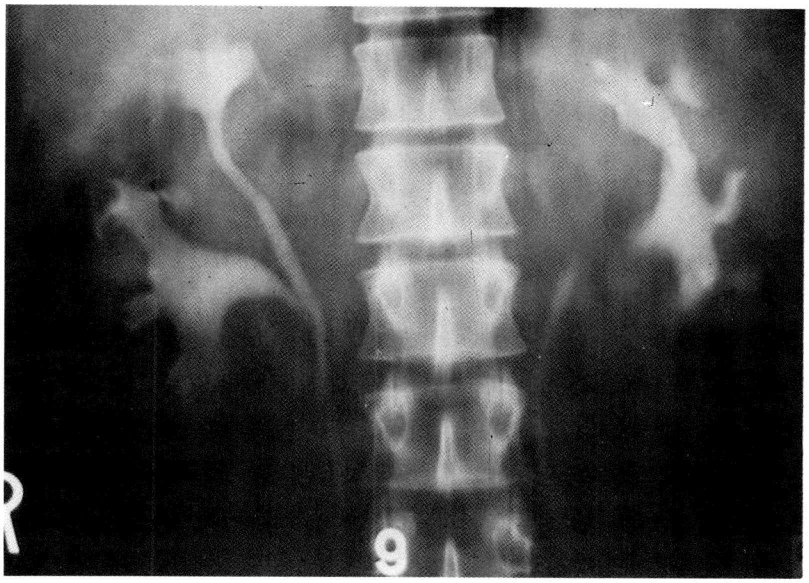

140

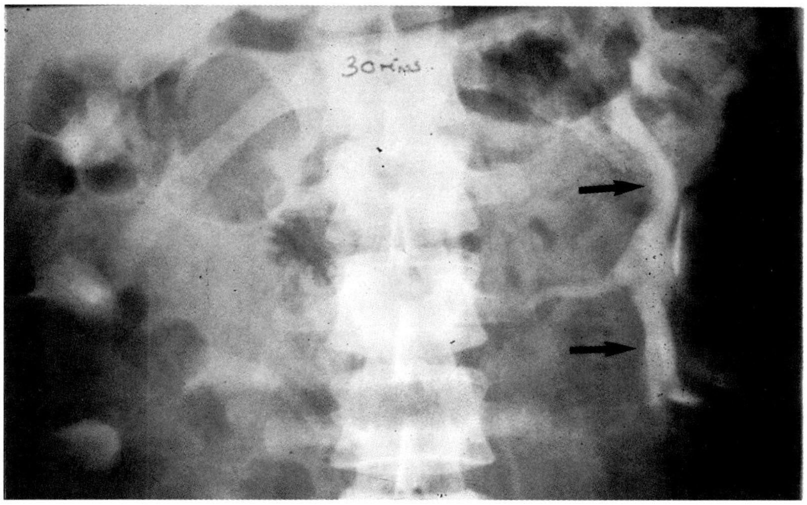

139, 140 Adult type polycystic disease is a progressive disorder. Shown here are an intravenous urogram (**139**) and a retrograde urogram (**140**) separated by six years. Serum creatinine was normal at the time of the initial investigation but had risen to three times normal six years later. Note progressive distortion of the calyces with increasing replacement of the renal parenchyma by the cysts (arrows, **140**).

141

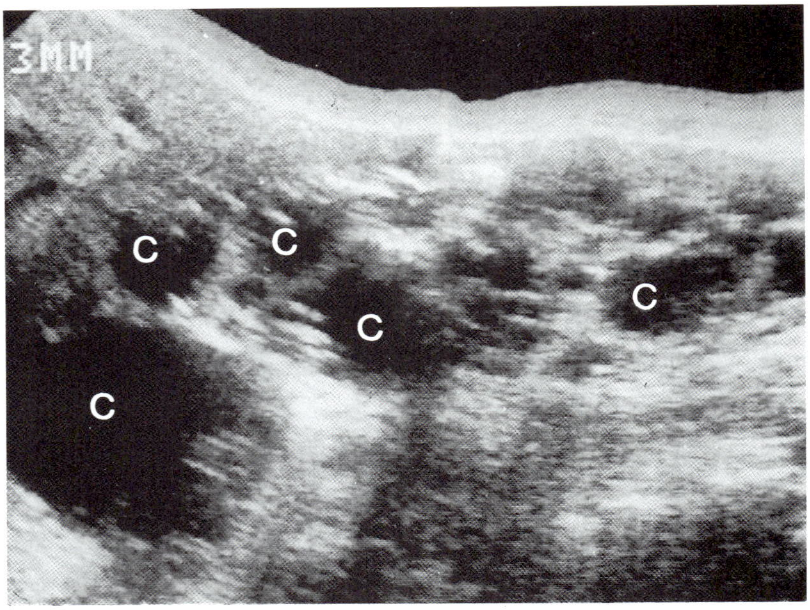

141 Renal ultrasound demonstrates multiple cysts in a large polycystic kidney.

142

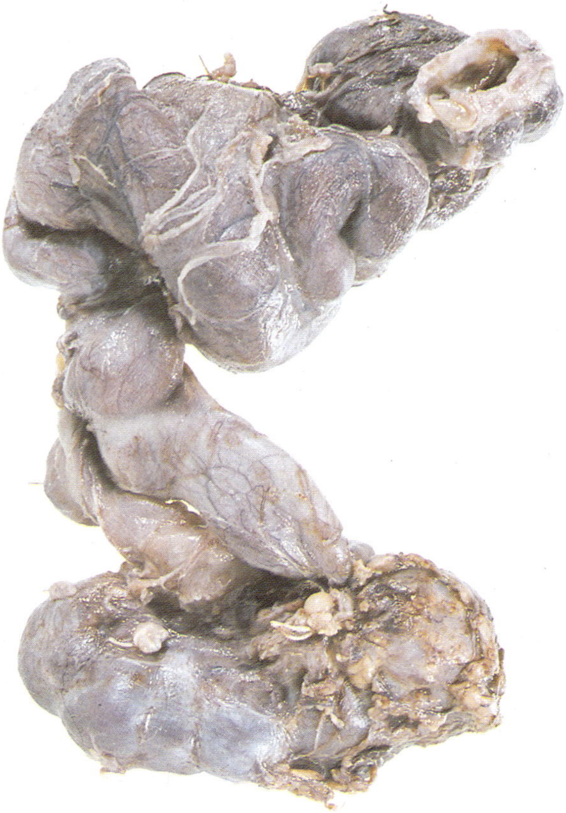

142 Macroscopic appearance of dysplastic kidney removed from an infant of six months. There is a markedly dilated and tortuous ureter with a small deformed kidney containing abnormal and distorted calyces. On microscopic examination the renal parenchyma had radial seams secondary to reflux and also contained abnormally differentiated/developed tissues.

Endocrine causes of hypertension

Hypertension may occur as part of the clinical presentation of many endocrine syndromes. Such patients represent less than 1% of all hypertensives. Hypertension may be the presenting feature, as in Conn's syndrome and phaeochromocytoma, or part of a varied clinical spectrum, as in Cushing's syndrome and acromegaly.

Cushing's syndrome

In 1832 the Baltimore surgeon, Harvey Cushing, described a syndrome characterized by trunkal obesity, fatigue, weakness, amenorrhoea, hirsuitism, abdominal striae, glycosuria, oedema, osteoporosis, and hypertension. This is now known as Cushing's syndrome. Hypertension is one of the most common features of this condition, and occurs in 80% of these patients. If left untreated, it may cause congestive heart failure and death. As with hypertension of other endocrine causes, the longer it is present, the less likely it is to regress when the underlying cause is treated. The hypertension is one of the causative factors in the accelerated atherosclerosis seen in this condition. It has become apparent in the last few decades that Cushing's syndrome may arise in several ways. Mostly, it is due to bilateral adrenal hyperplasia, the predominant feature being the excessive production of glucocorticoids and androgens. This is caused by ACTH-secreting tumours arising in the pituitary gland (Cushing's disease), or from non-endocrine sites (ectopic ACTH secretion). Up to 20% of cases are due to primary adrenal adenomas or carcinomas. This condition is more frequent in women and presents in the middle third of life.

43

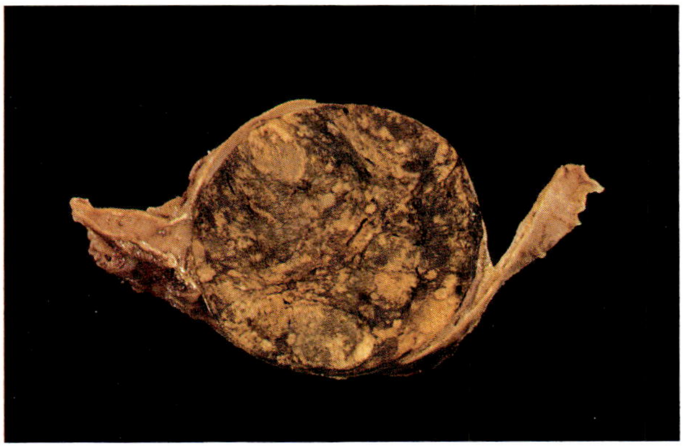

144

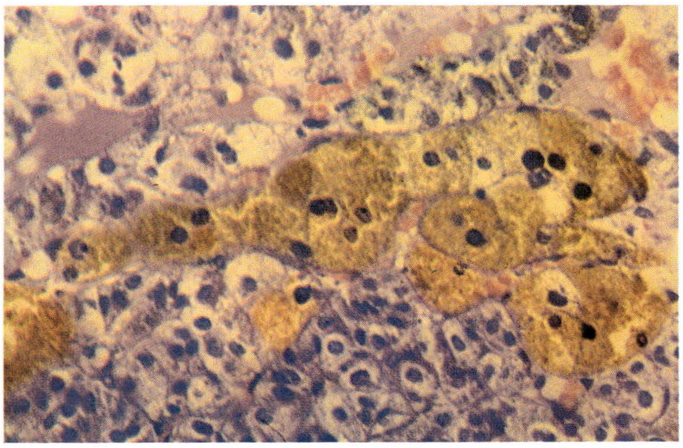

143 Cortical adenoma of the adrenal gland in a patient with Cushing's syndrome. There is a 3 cm spherical tumour which has a dark brown and yellow cut surface. The remainder of the adrenal cortex is thin and atrophic.

144 Histology of the adrenal gland in Cushing's syndrome; this cortical adenoma contains a varied cell content. There are pale staining large cells rich in sudanophilic lipid, other large cells with abundant brown granules, and an area of small cells compactly arranged.

145

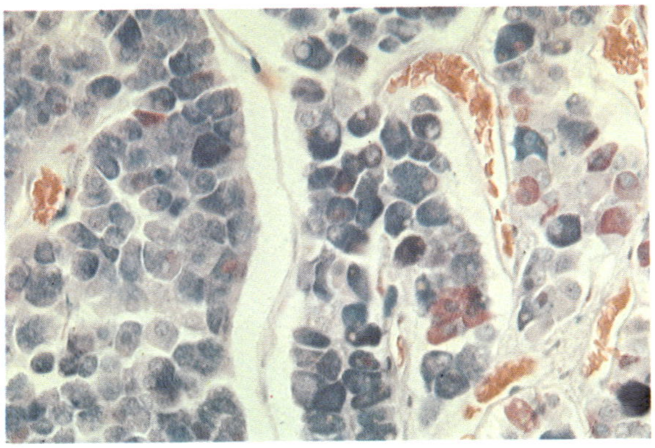

145 Basophil adenoma of the pituitary gland in a patient with Cushing's disease.

146

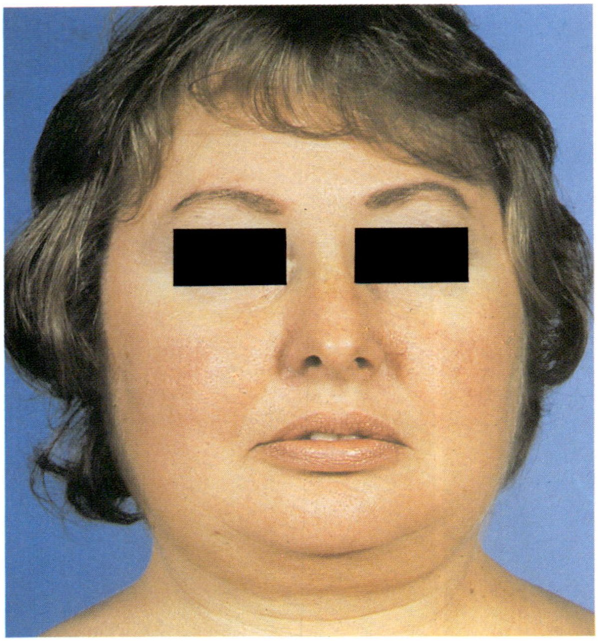

14

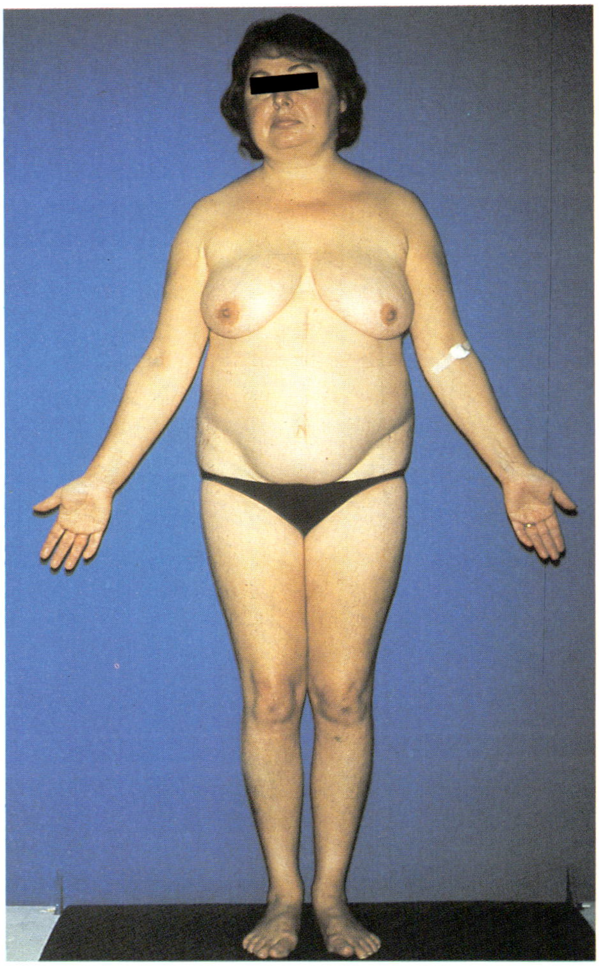

146–151 Cushing's syndrome patients have a typical body appearance with a moon face, central obesity and slender limbs with loss of proximal muscle strength and bulk. Glucose intolerance occurs in up to 20% of patients and hypertension occurs in most. Androgen excess frequently presents as hirsuitism, amenorrhoea, clitoromegaly, and deepening of the voice. The moon facial appearance and the deep purple abdominal striae are typical of Cushing's syndrome and may be seen in both mild (**146, 147**) and severe cases (**148, 149**). Exogenous corticosteroid use is also an important cause of hypertension and may lead to Cushingoid features (**150, 151**).

48

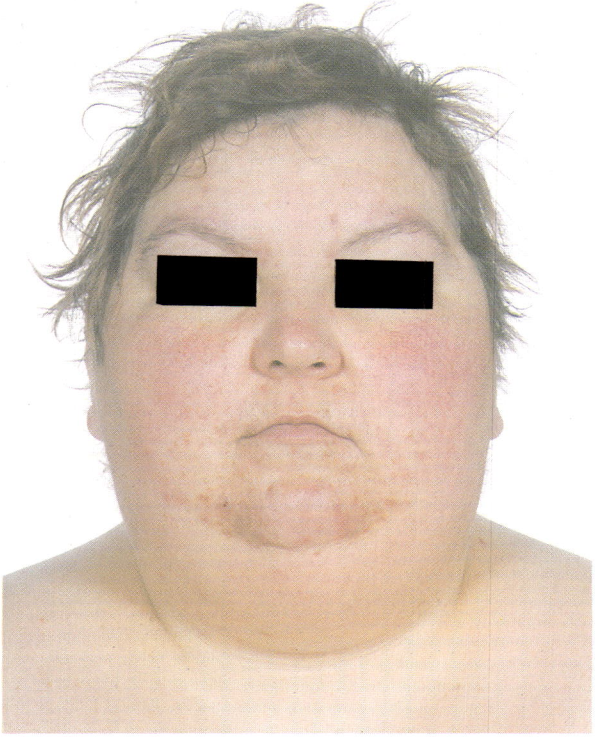

149

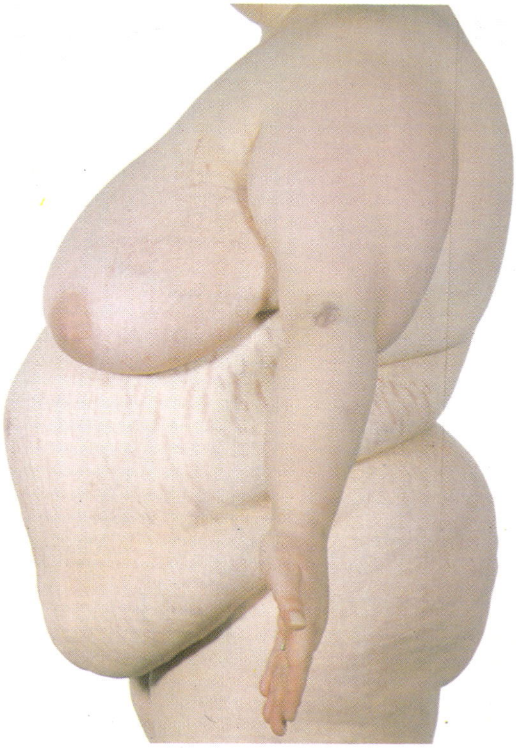

50

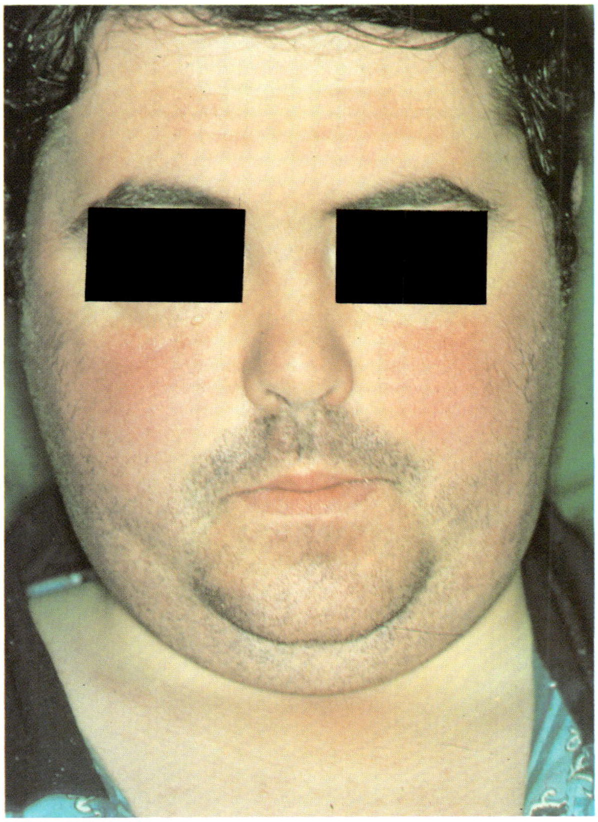

151

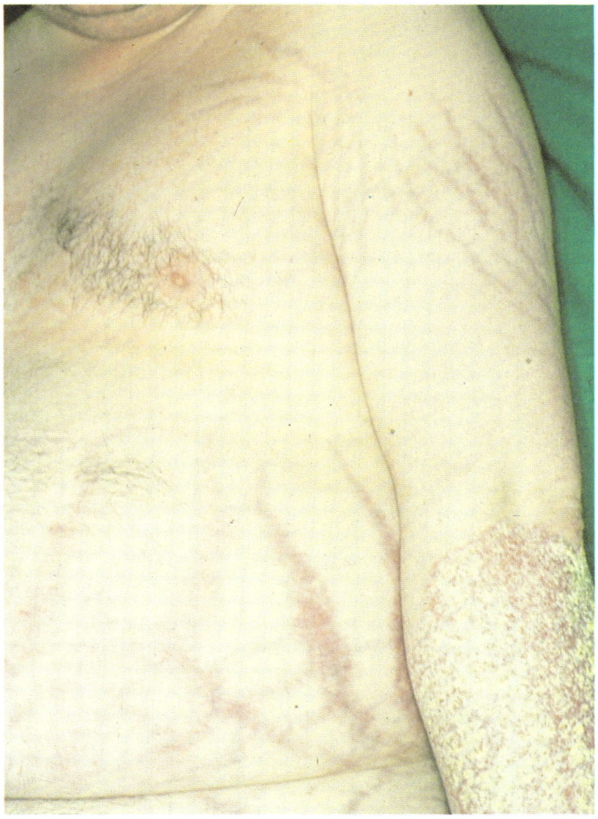

152

	Adrenocortical hyperplasia		Adrenocortical tumour	
	Pituitary dependent	**Ectopic ACTH**	**Carcinoma**	**Adenoma**
PLASMA CORTISOL				
MORNING	↑	↑	↑	↑
EVENING	↑	↑	↑	↑
after 2 mg dexamethasone	← NO SUPPRESSION →			
after 8 mg dexamethasone	SUPPRESSION	← NO SUPPRESSION →		
URINARY CORTISOL	↑	↑↑	↑↑	↑
PLASMA ACTH	↑	↑	↓	↓

152 The laboratory diagnosis of Cushing's syndrome may be established by the dexamethasone suppression test. This demonstrates the lack of appropriate suppression of cortisol secretion when 2 or 8 mg of dexamethasone is given at bedtime with measurements of early morning cortisol. Measurement of the urinary free cortisol level may also be a useful screening test. Measurement of plasma ACTH may be useful in differentiating Cushing's syndrome and disease.

153 CT scan of the abdomen showing bilateral adrenal hyperplasia (arrows) in Cushing's disease.

153

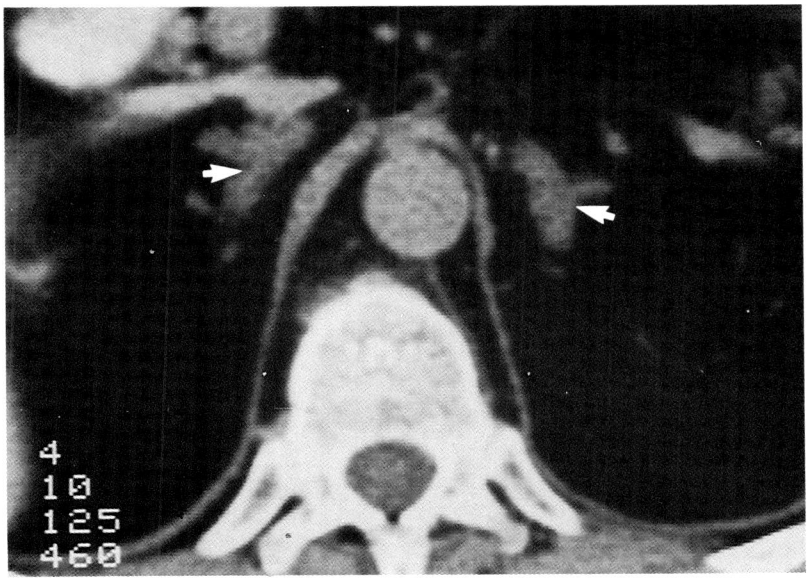

54

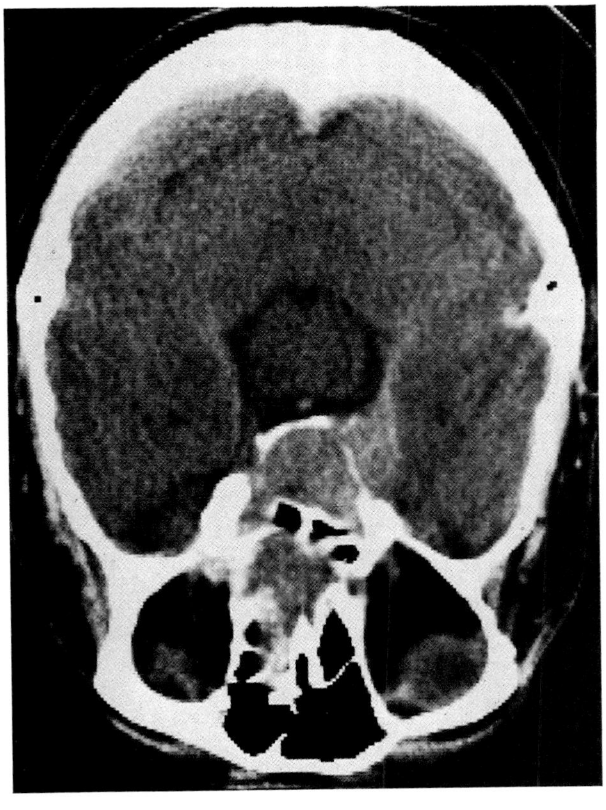

155

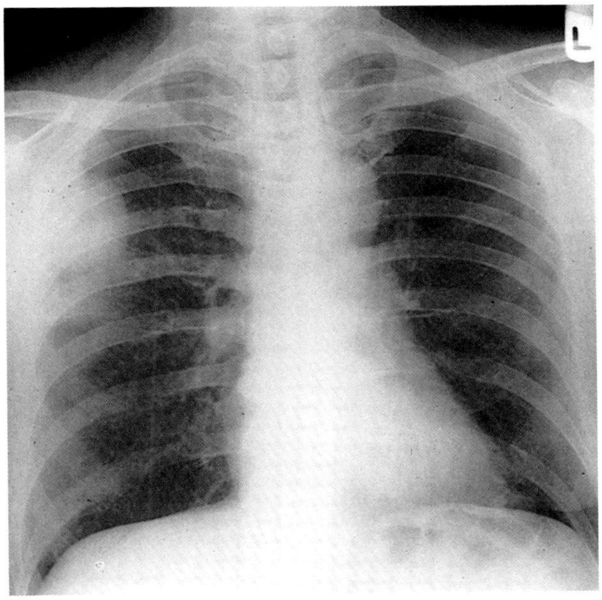

155 Cushing's syndrome may be caused by ACTH secretion sites other than the pituitary. Ectopic ACTH syndromes may arise from a variety of sites, the most common being bronchial carcinomas, as seen in this example of a solitary lesion of the right upper lobe. Resection of such tumours, if complete, will lead to regression of Cushing's syndrome.

154 CT scan of the pituitary fossa from a patient with Cushing's disease. There is a large mass in the area of the pituitary that is an ACTH-secreting tumour. Cushing's disease, with over-production of ACTH by the pituitary, occurs in two-thirds of the patients with Cushing's syndrome. The pituitary adenoma may be quite small and discrete.

Conn's syndrome (primary aldosteronism)

Conn's syndrome is a rare cause of hypertension that was first recognized in 1954, and is due to the hypersecretion of aldosterone from an adrenal adenoma. It is associated with hypertension, hypokalaemia, and a metabolic alkalosis. Glucose intolerance and polyuria may also be present.

There are few clinical findings to suggest the presence of Conn's syndrome and to distinguish it from essential hypertension. The aldosteronism increases sodium reabsorption and potassium excretion. This leads to hypernatraemia and expands the plasma volume, causing hypertension and suppressing the renin angiotensin system. Increased potassium excretion leads to hypokalaemia, muscle weakness, metabolic alkalosis and polyuria. Following the stage of increased plasma volume, peripheral vascular resistance rises. High levels of atrial naturetic peptide are also present.

Hypertension in Conn's syndrome may be severe and develop into a malignant phase. Patients with Conn's syndrome have an increased risk of developing vascular complications of hypertension, such as stroke or myocardial infarction. The diagnosis should be considered when hypertension and hypokalaemia coexist. Rarely will the patient be normokalaemic and the diagnosis is likely to be missed. Urinary potassium excretion will be increased, and the diagnosis confirmed by the presence of suppressed plasma renin activity and elevated serum aldosterone levels (this assay is not widely available). The tumour may be imaged directly with abdominal ultrasound or CT scanning.

156

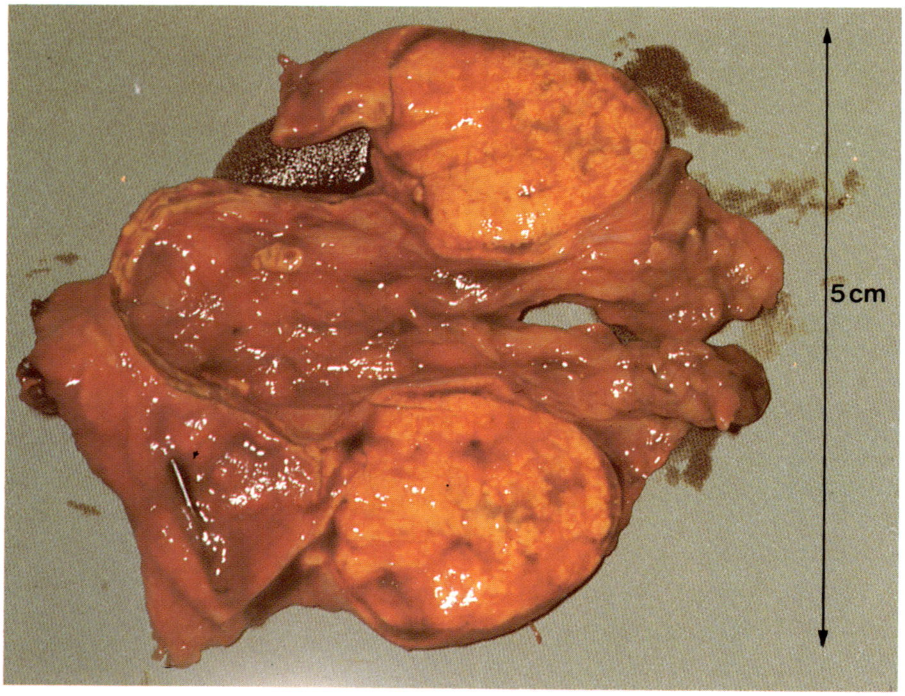

156 Gross pathology in Conn's syndrome showing a typical adrenal adenoma (cut).

157

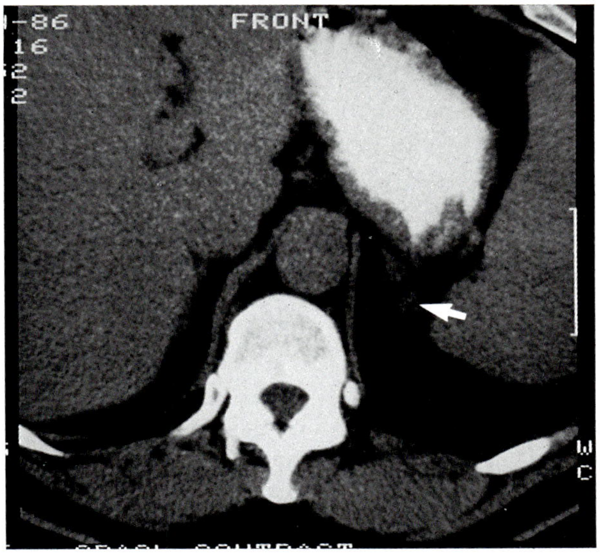

157 Abdominal CT scan with contrast enhancement showing a suprarenal mass posterior to the adrenal gland (arrow): this tumour was aldosterone-producing in a hypertensive patient. Removal of the tumour led to a reduction in blood pressure.

158

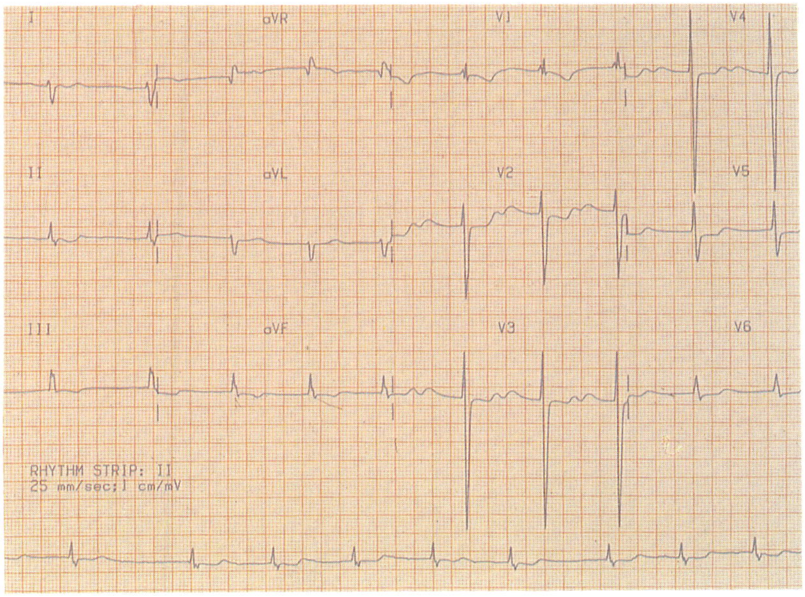

158 Electrocardiogram in Conn's syndrome. This shows the typical features of hypokalaemia with a significant U-wave, ST segment depression, T-wave inversion and prolonged QT interval.

Phaeochromocytoma

Hypertension may be caused by the increased secretion of catecholamines from an adrenal or extra-adrenal neoplasm, a phaeochromocytoma. The association of paroxysmal hypertension and an adrenal medullary tumour was first reported in 1922. This condition is characterized by dramatic symptoms and marked variations in blood pressure.

Paroxysmal hypertension may be provoked by a number of stresses, including anaesthesia and injection of angiographic contrast media. Histamine, caffeine, nicotine, beta-blockers and tricyclic antidepressants may all lead to paroxysms of hypertension, or, occasionally, hypotension. Sudden episodes of headache, sweating, pallor, palpitation, nervousness, nausea and vomiting, pain in the chest or abdomen may also be presenting features. These paroxysms may be incorrectly ascribed to menopausal hot flushes or psychological causes. The catecholamine secretion may lead to direct myocardial damage. Stroke and hypertensive crises with encephalopathy and retinal haemorrhages may occur.

Phaeochromocytomas may arise wherever the sympathagonia from the primitive neural crest comes to rest. Of these tumours, 90% arise in the adrenal medulla, of which 10% are bilateral and another 10% are malignant. Phaeochromocytomas may appear in Sipple syndrome in association with medullary carcinoma of the thyroid. Phaeochromocytoma may be a familial condition and may be found in patients with neurofibromatosis and hypertension.

The screening test for this condition is a 24-hour urinary estimation of VMA (vanillyl mandelic acid) or metanephrine. The measurement of lying and standing plasma catecholamine levels will usually confirm the diagnosis. In a hypertensive patient with a raised catecholamine level, the tumour may be localized by ultrasound, CT scanning, or magnetic resonance imaging. Meta Iodo Benzyl Guanidine (MIBG) scanning and venous sampling may also be used to localize a tumour.

159

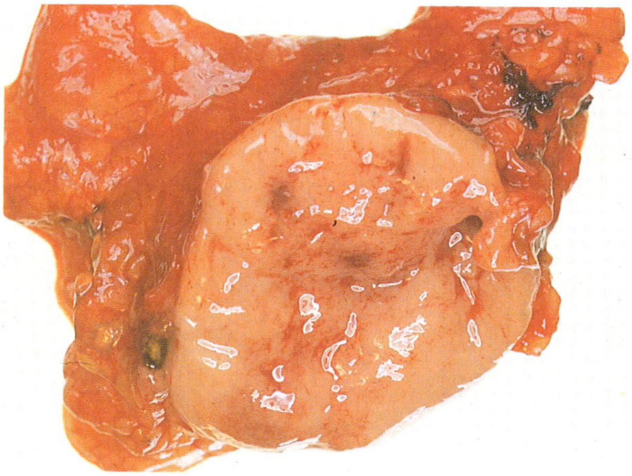

160

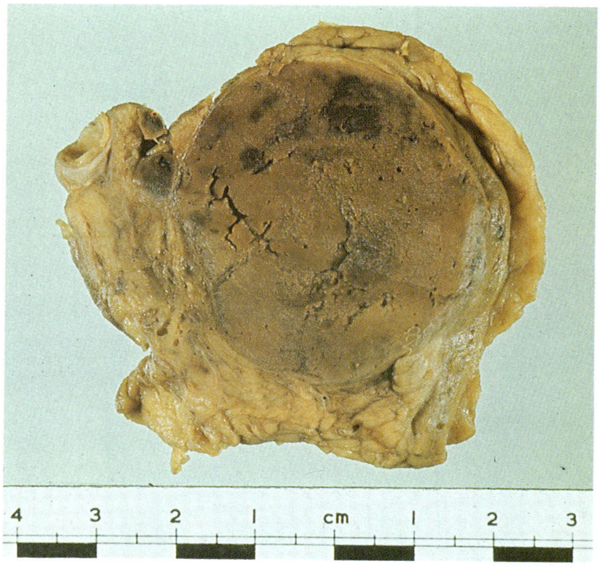

159, 160 Gross pathology of a fresh (**159**) and formalin fixed (**160**) adrenal phaeochromocytoma.

61a

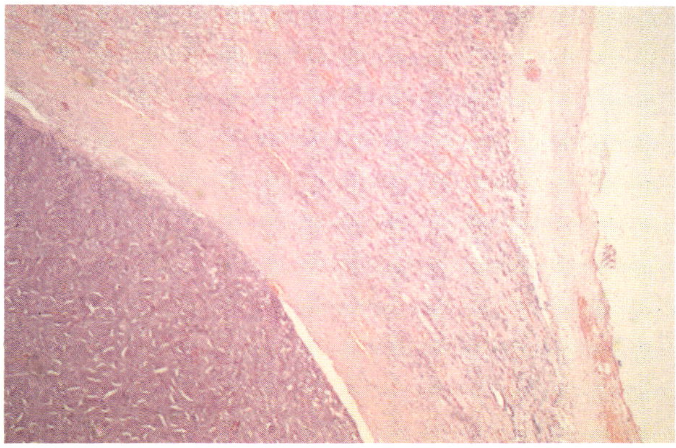

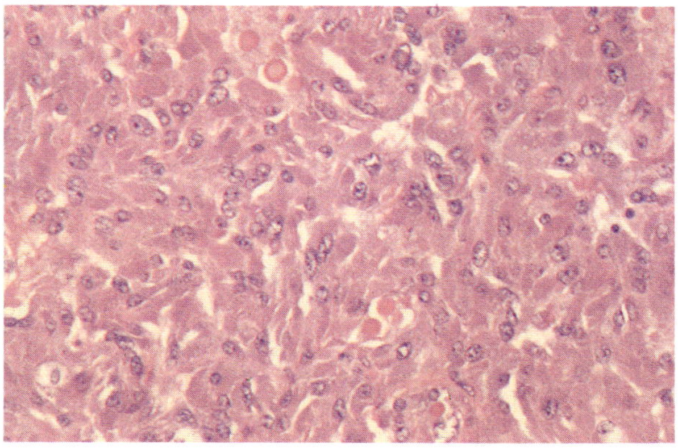

161b

161a, 161b Histology of the example in **159**. At low power the distinction between the dark staining tumour and normal adrenal tissue can be seen (**161a**). At higher power the alveolar arrangement of cells is seen to be similar to those of the normal medulla (**161b**). They may have abundant eosinophilic cytoplasm, and mitoses are rare in this benign tumour.

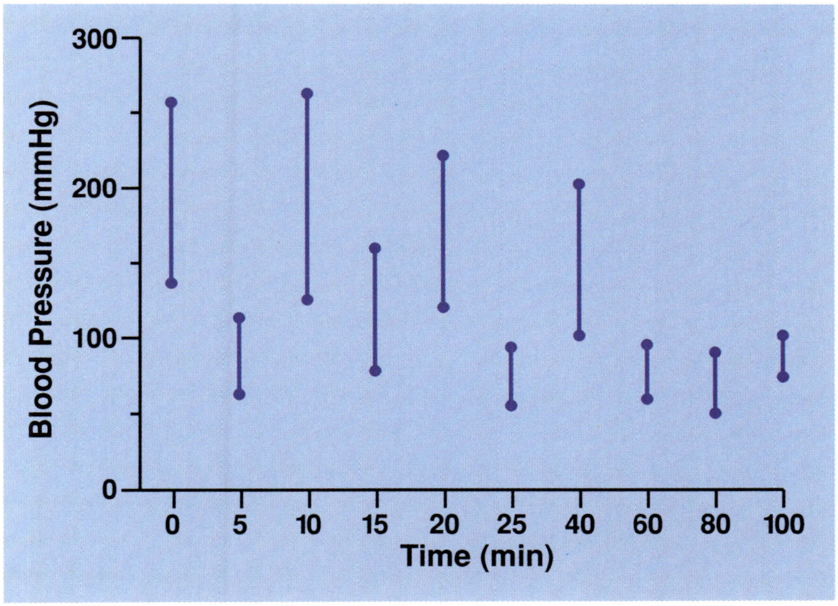

162

162 Blood pressure response following endoscopy in a patient with unsuspected phaeochromocytoma.

163

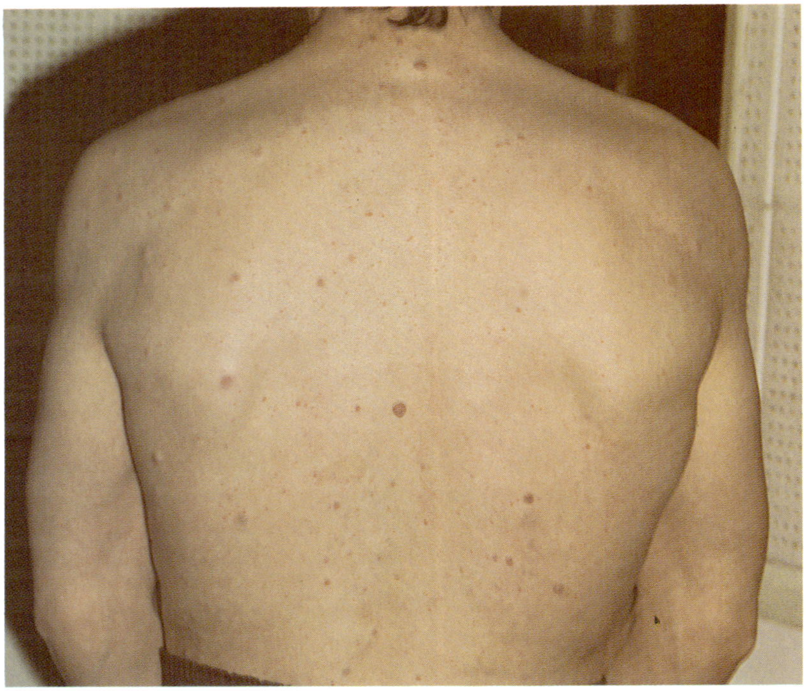

164

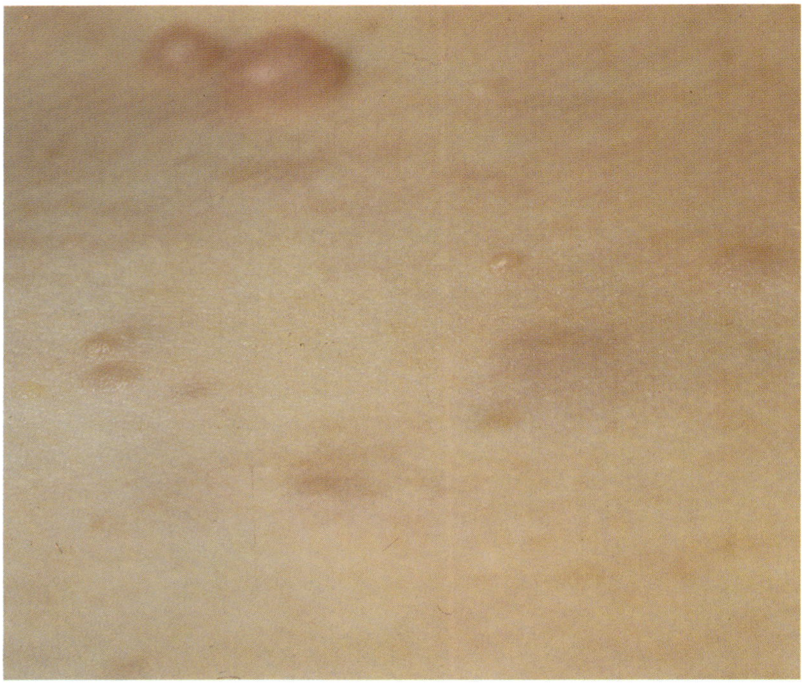

163, 164 Back of a patient with neurofibromatosis and hypertension. There is evidence of scoliosis and cutaneous neurofibromata.

165, 166 Postero-anterior and lateral chest X-ray in a patient with neurofibromatosis. A huge neurofibroma originates from the spinal canal and into the right upper thorax, causing kyphoscoliosis.

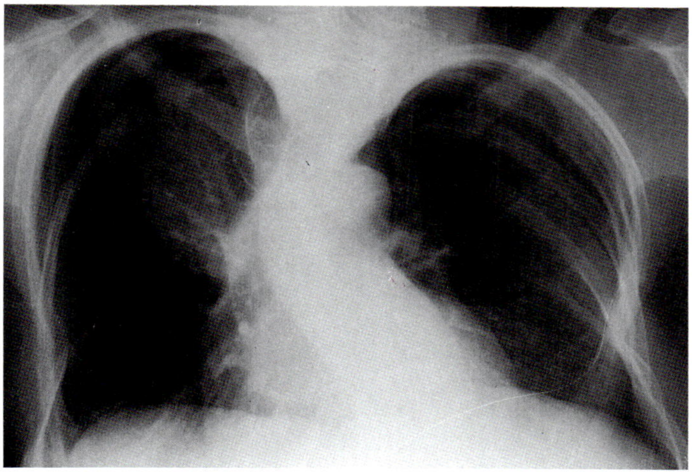

165

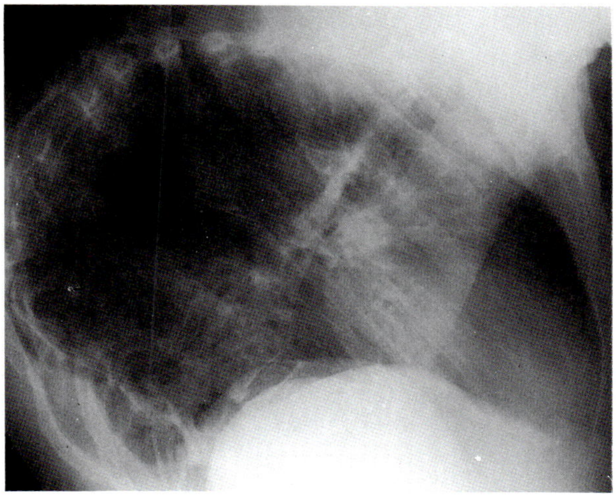

166

167 Pentolinium suppression test in a patient with a markedly elevated serum adrenaline level. Administration of pentolinium (P) fails to return the adrenaline level to within the normal range, shown here as the hatched line, indicating an autonomous source of adrenaline production.

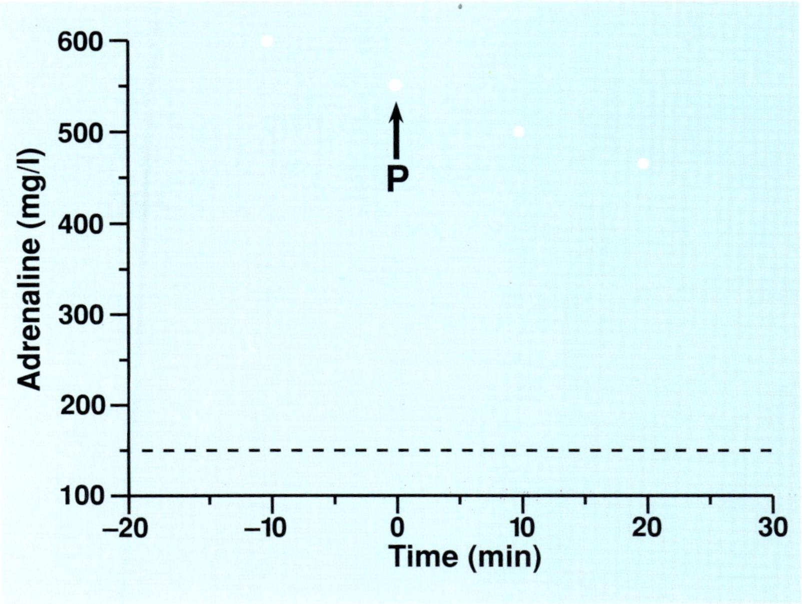

167

168

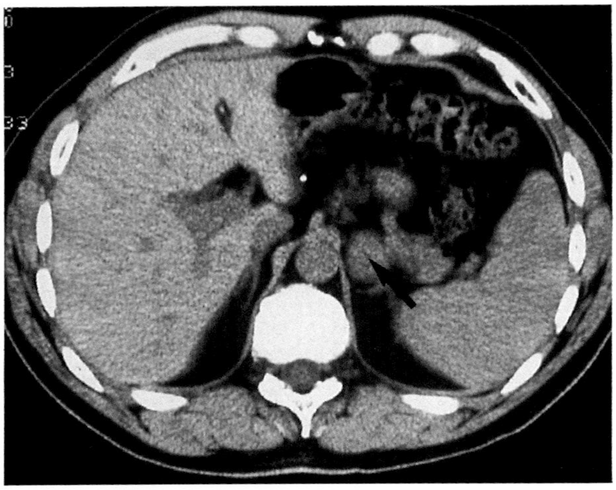

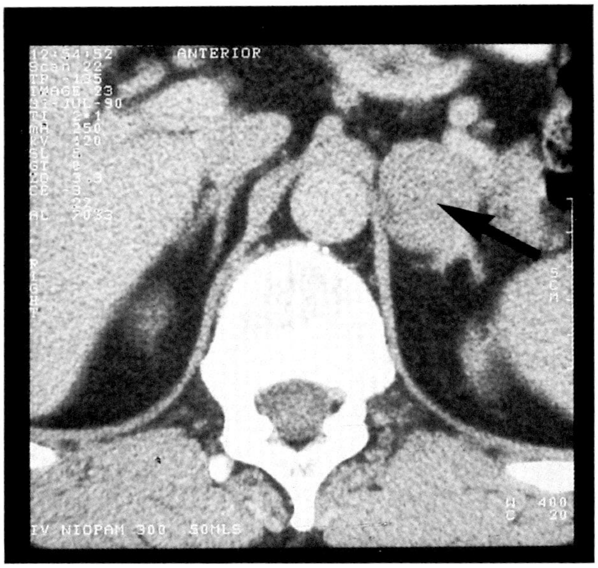

169

168, 169 CT scans of the abdomen in a patient with a 3–4 cm phaeochromocytoma in the left adrenal gland (arrows), the pathology of which is shown in **159**.

170

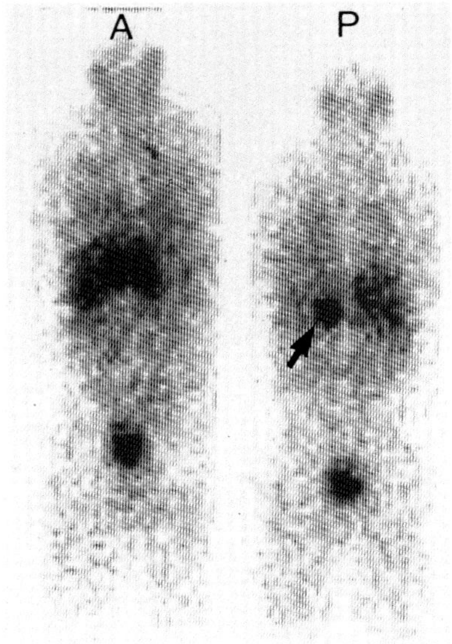

17

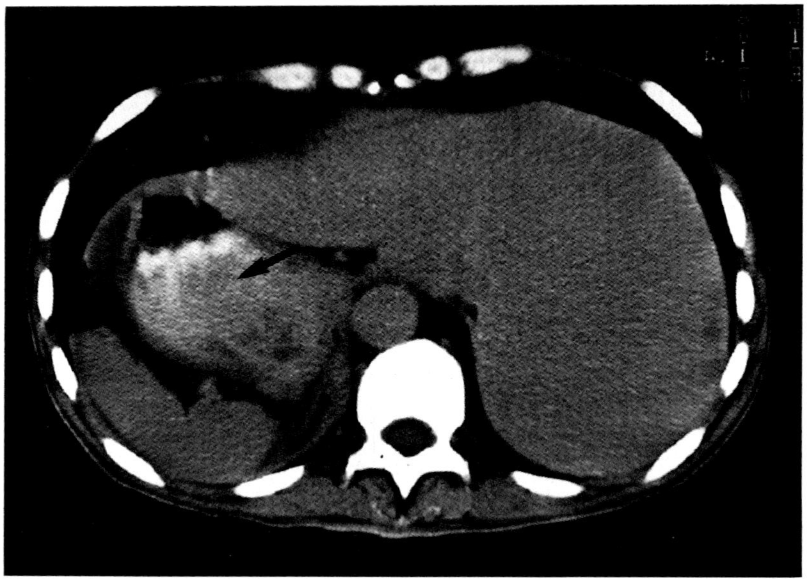

170 MIBG scan with increased uptake in the area of the left adrenal gland (arrow) in the patient shown in **168** and **169**. There is normal uptake in the liver and bladder.

171 CT scan of the abdomen in a hypertensive patient with a huge tumour anterior to the spleen which histologically was shown to be a phaeochromocytoma.

172

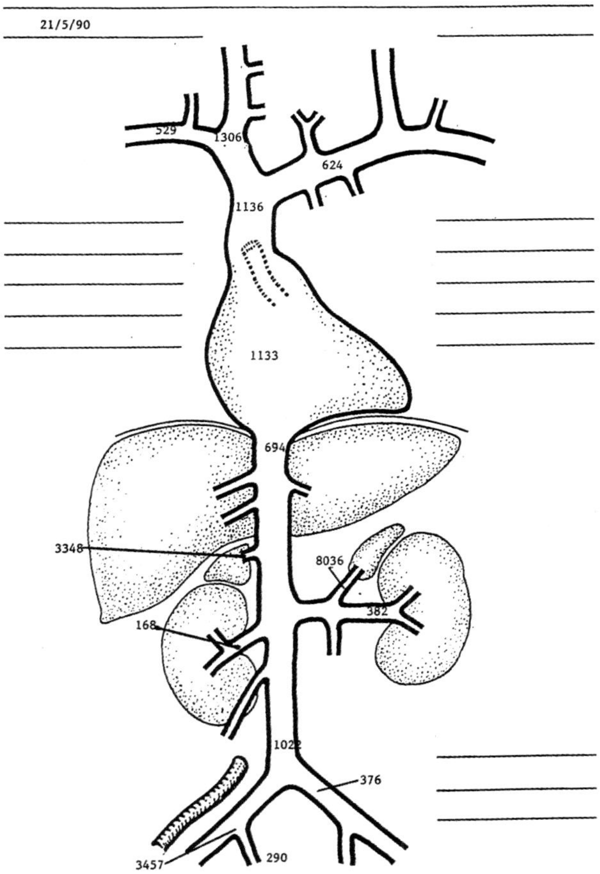

173

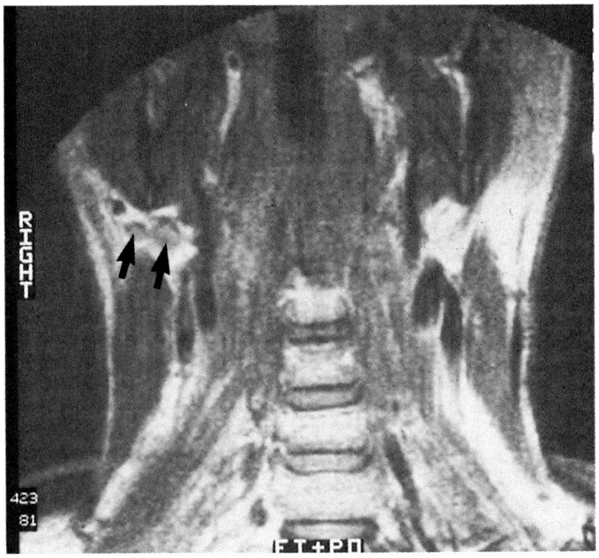

173 MR scan, coronal section through the neck, demonstrating two masses at the level of the carotid bifurcation in the patient in **172**.

172 Venous sampling with abnormally raised adrenaline levels in the right internal iliac and the right brachiocephalic veins. This indicates there is a phaeochromocytoma in the areas drained by these veins.

174 Electrocardiogram in phaeochromocytoma showing deep symmetrical T-wave inversion with a small increase in QRS voltage. Such changes may reflect the catecholamine cardiomyopathy of this condition.

174

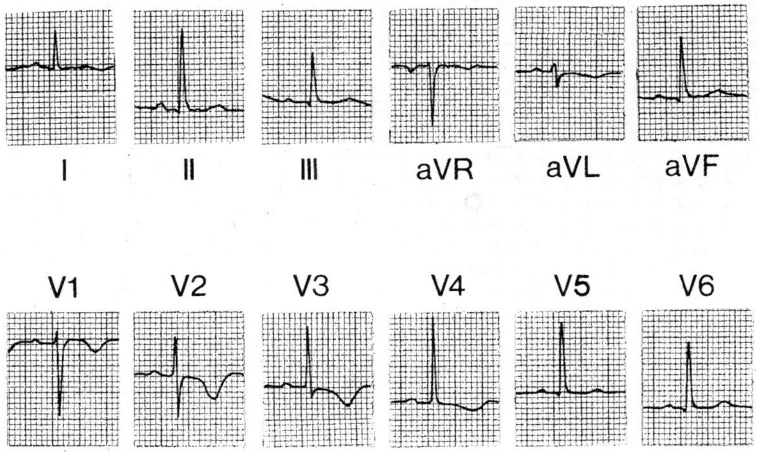

Acromegaly

Hypertension is the most common cardiovascular manifestation of acromegaly, occurring in 15–50% of patients. Acromegalic patients with hypertension tend to be older and have a longer disease duration than those with normal blood pressure.

The underlying mechanisms involved are unclear, but the hypertension is usually mild, uncomplicated, and responds quite readily to the usual antihypertensive medication. Growth hormone, which may be the hypertensive agent, originates from the anterior pituitary gland and is one of many hormones secreted by this organ. Acromegaly is almost invariably the result of a growth hormone producing chromophobic or eosinophilic pituitary adenoma, although rarely it may be secondary to ectopic production of growth hormone or somatotrophin-releasing hormone.

The disease is characteristically slowly progressive, with signs and symptoms often predating diagnosis by many years. The clinical findings are broad, spade-like hands and feet, which result from the growth of connective tissue, muscle and bone. The growth of the mandible, frontal ridges, nose, and ears are all prominent features. Osteoarthritis is common, along with generalized organomegaly. Metabolic abnormalities of carbohydrate metabolism are a common consequence of chronic overproduction of growth hormone. Most patients have a state of insulin resistance with high serum insulin levels, though clinical diabetes mellitus is present in only 10%. The acromegaly leads to a number of cardiac manifestations, including cardiac enlargement, hypertension, premature coronary artery disease, heart failure and cardiac arrhythmias. It remains unclear whether a specific heart muscle disease due to acromegaly exists, or if this is just a manifestation of hypertension, premature coronary artery disease and diabetes.

175

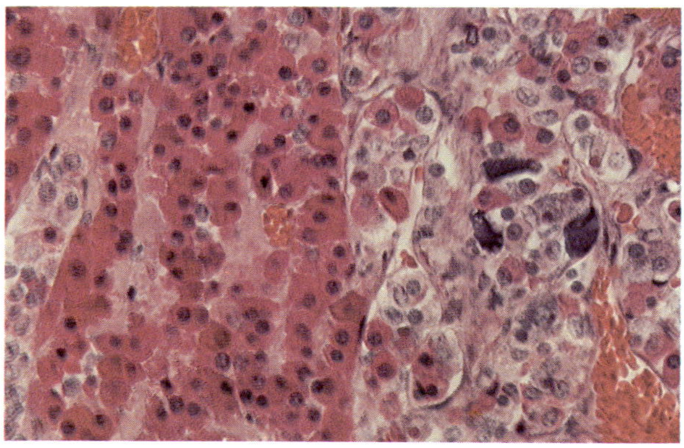

175 Pituitary gland in a patient with acromegaly containing an eosinophilic adenoma. The stain used (eosin Isamine blue) shows eosinophils as red, basophils as blue-purple, and chromophobes as pale grey or unstained.

176

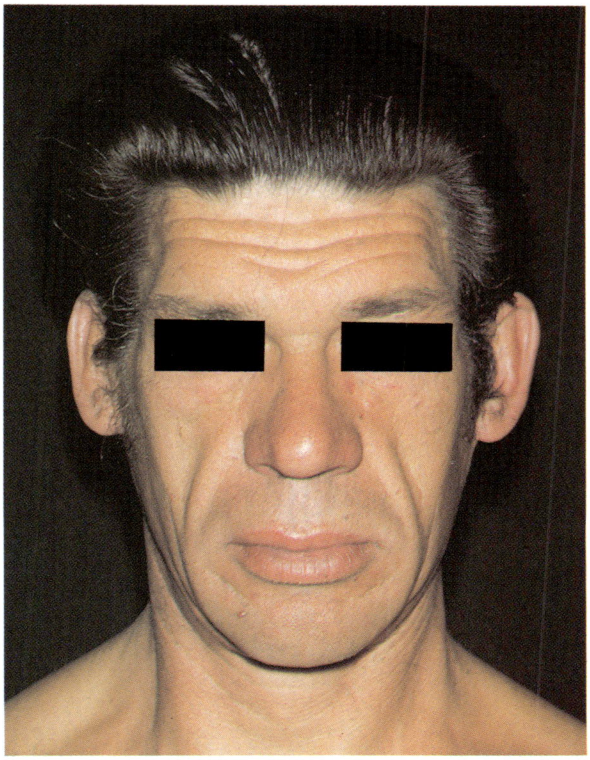

177

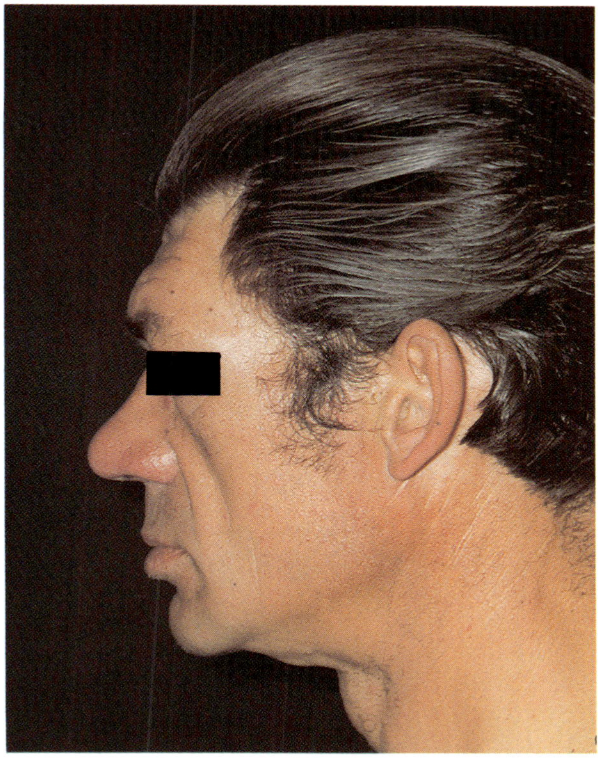

178

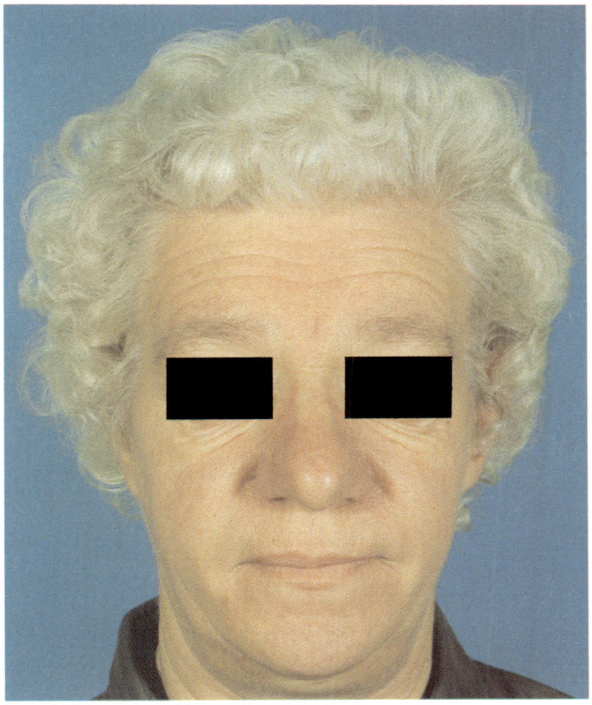

179

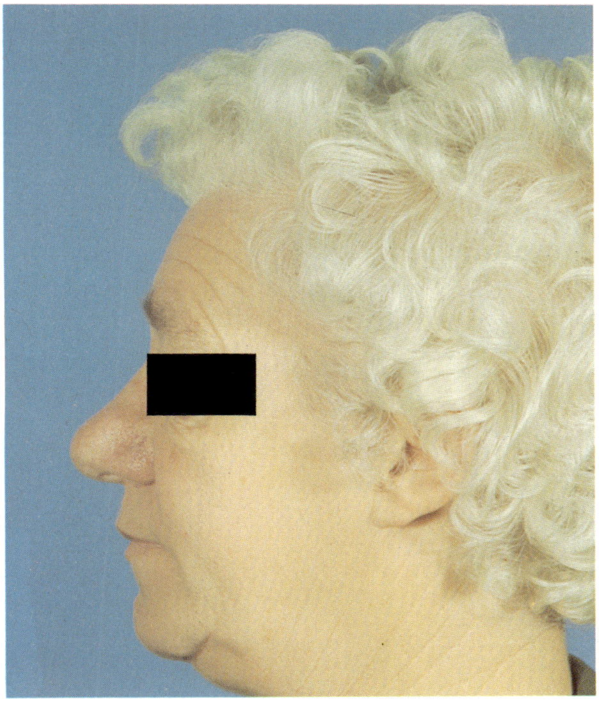

176–179 The typical facies of acromegaly in a mild (**176, 177**) and a more severe (**178, 179**) case. There is a prominent mandible with overgrowth of the frontal ridges. Connective tissue is thickened. It is not uncommon for the patient to complain of increasing hat size.

180

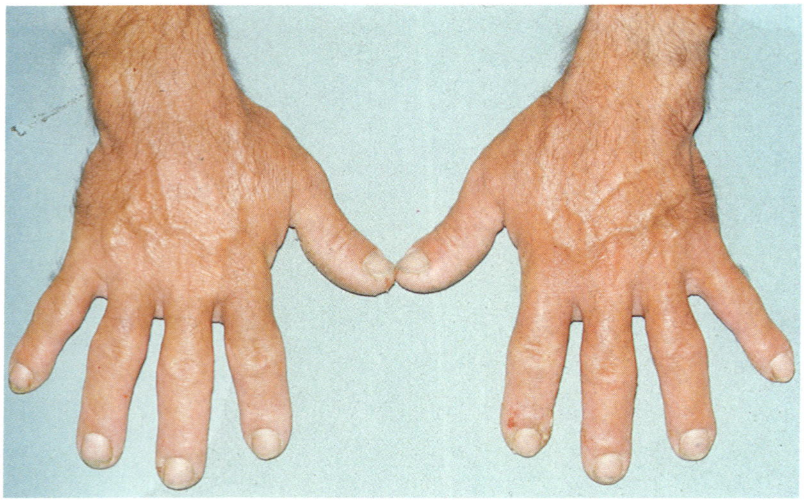

180–182 The hands in acromegaly may be minimally involved (**180**) or broad and spade-like (**181**). The feet may be similarly involved (**182**).

181

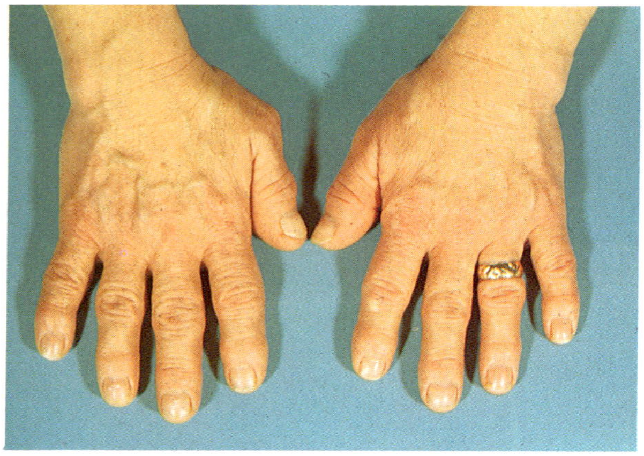

182

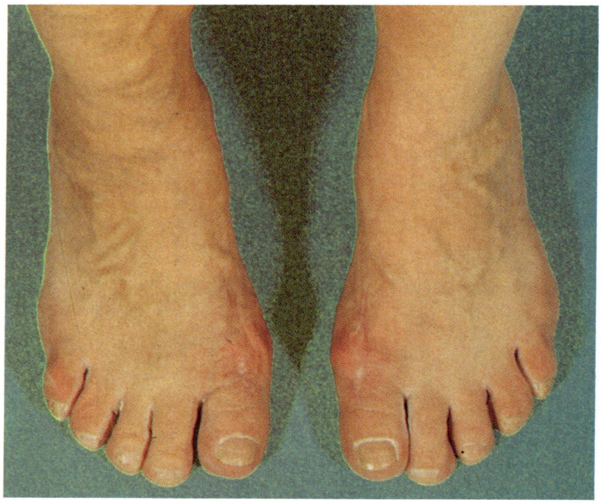

183

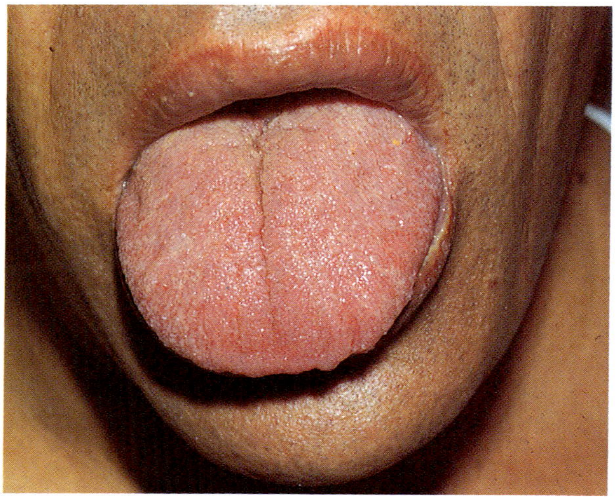

183 Enlargement of the tongue is frequently seen in acromegaly and is one of the differential diagnoses of macroglossia.

184 Overgrowth of the mandible leads to separation of the teeth.

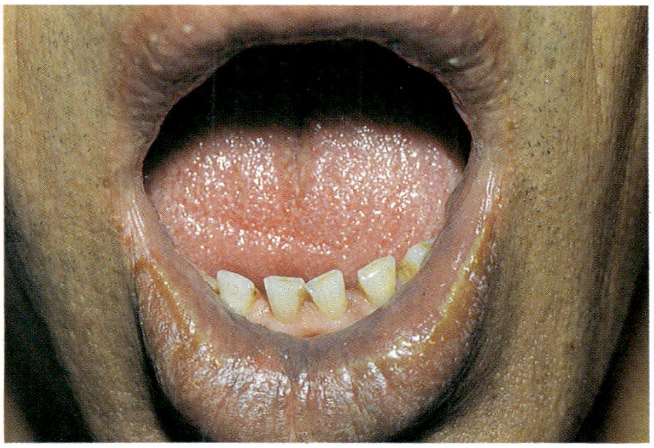

184

185 Lateral skull radiograph in a patient with acromegaly showing enlargement of the pituitary fossa due to an adenoma (arrows).

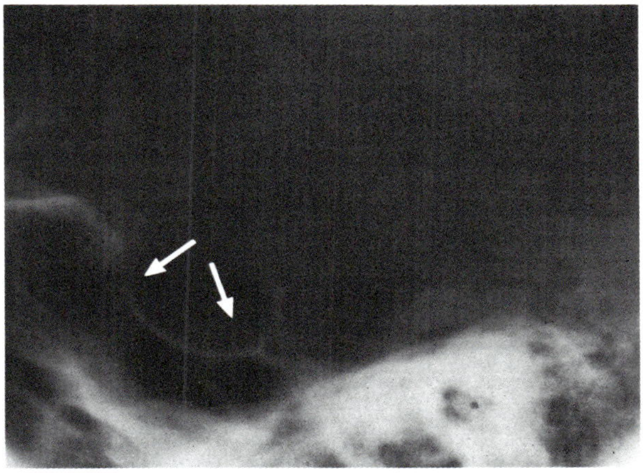

185

186 Various radiological findings are commonly found in acromegaly but are not pathognomonic, including thickening of the heel pad.

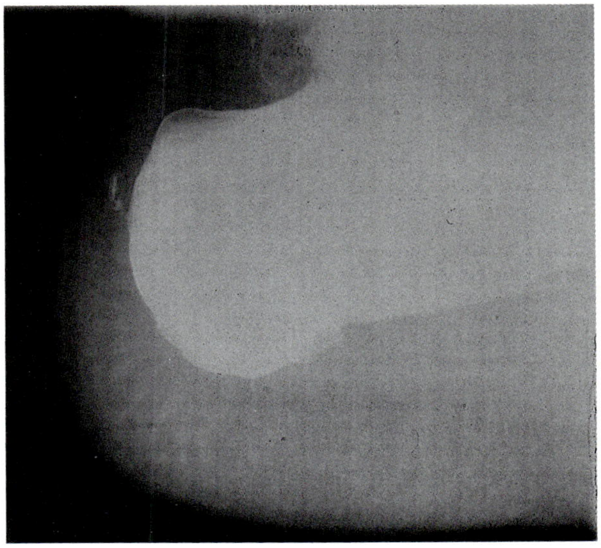

186

187

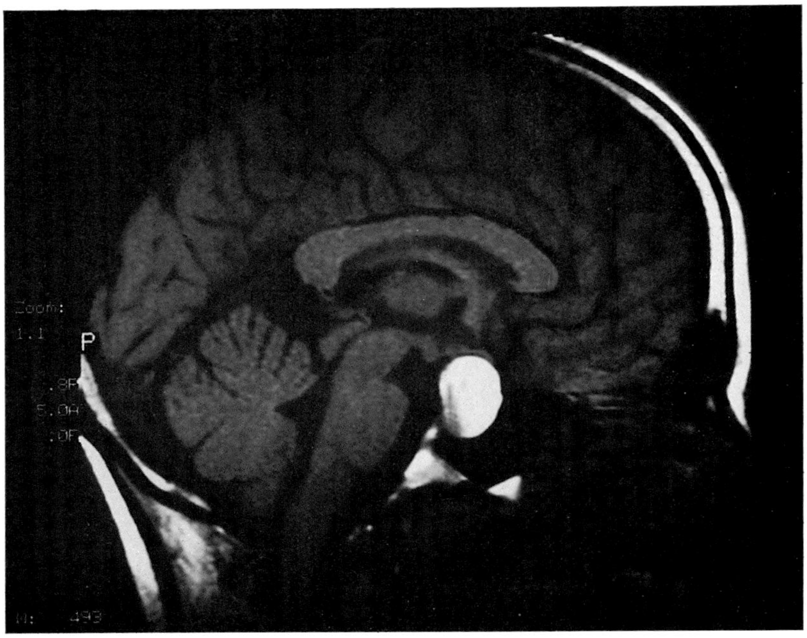

188

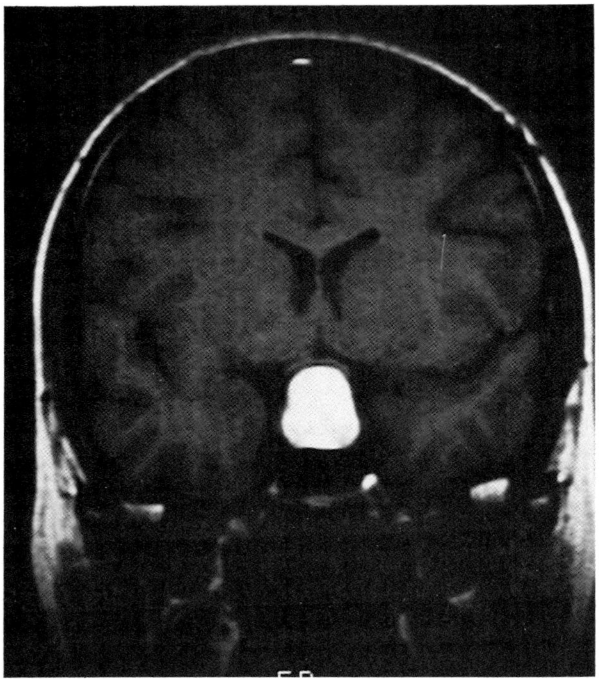

18

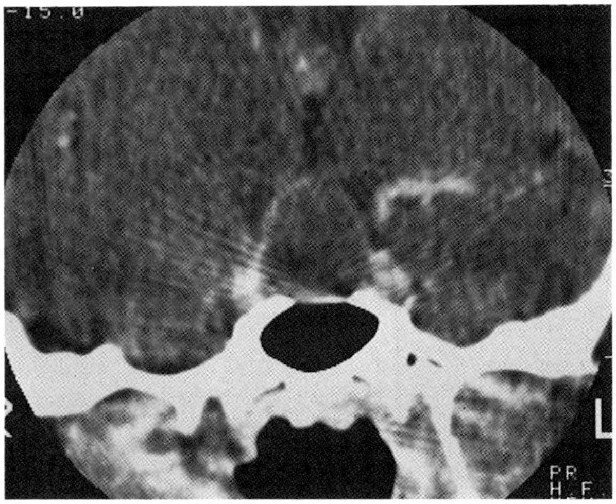

187–189 CT scans showing enlargement of the pituitary due to an adenoma. This is a large adenoma seen with contrast enhancement in the lateral and coronal views (**187**, **188**) and without enhancement in a specialized pituitary view (**189**).

Vascular causes of hypertension

Renovascular hypertension

In 1934, Goldblatt produced hypertension in a dog by clipping one renal artery. The mechanism of this hypertension is increased renin release from the ischaemic kidney, induced by diminished perfusion pressure in the renal afferent arteriole. When renovascular hypertension leads to extensive nephrosclerosis in the contralateral kidney, a second mechanism for hypertension may evolve. At this stage, relief of the renal artery stenosis may not reduce the hypertension, as the contralateral kidney sustains the level of raised blood pressure.

Hypertension is due to renal artery stenosis in less than 2% of adults. The majority of renal artery stenosis is caused by atherosclerosis, and therefore the incidence of this condition rises with age. The highest prevalence of renal artery stenosis is among patients with severe and accelerated forms of hypertension. While 60% of renal artery stenosis is due to atherosclerosis, the remaining 40% is caused by fibroplastic diseases of the arteries. These non-atherosclerotic stenoses involve all layers of the renal artery, but the most common is medial fibroplasia. Suggestive features of renal artery stenosis include:

- The presence of a bruit in the abdomen, particularly if this is present in diastole and is heard lateral to the mid-line;
- Hypertension beginning before the age of 30;
- Hypertension after renal trauma;
- Difficult to control, rapidly accelerating hypertension;
- Deteriorating renal function after the use of an angiotensin converting enzyme inhibitor.

Two clinical forms of renal artery stenosis have been identified. The first occurs in older patients with atherosclerotic lesions who have high systolic blood pressure, and generalized arterial disease outside the kidney. These patients are quite likely to develop target organ damage. The second form includes patients with fibromuscular hyperplasia who are predominantly young, female, and less likely to develop cardiac disease, or have a family history of hypertension.

The confirmatory diagnostic test for renal artery stenosis is selective angiography. The diagnosis may be suspected by a unilateral delay in renal opacification on intravenous urography, isotopic renography, or digital subtraction angiography.

190

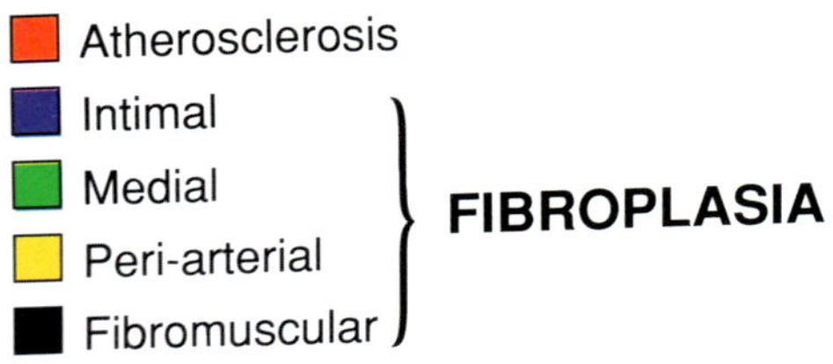

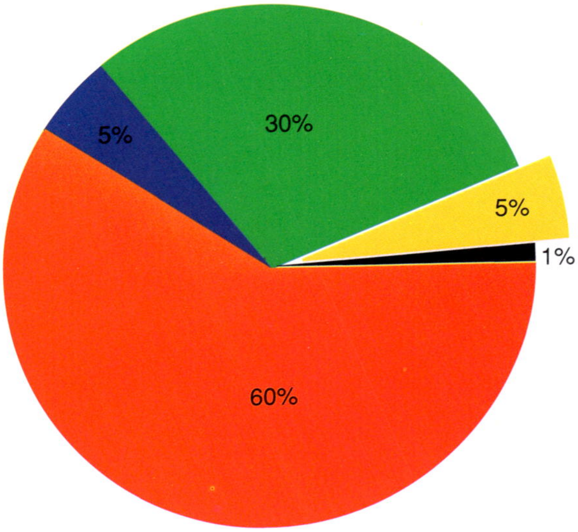

190 Pie chart showing the relative incidence of the various types of renal artery stenosis.

191

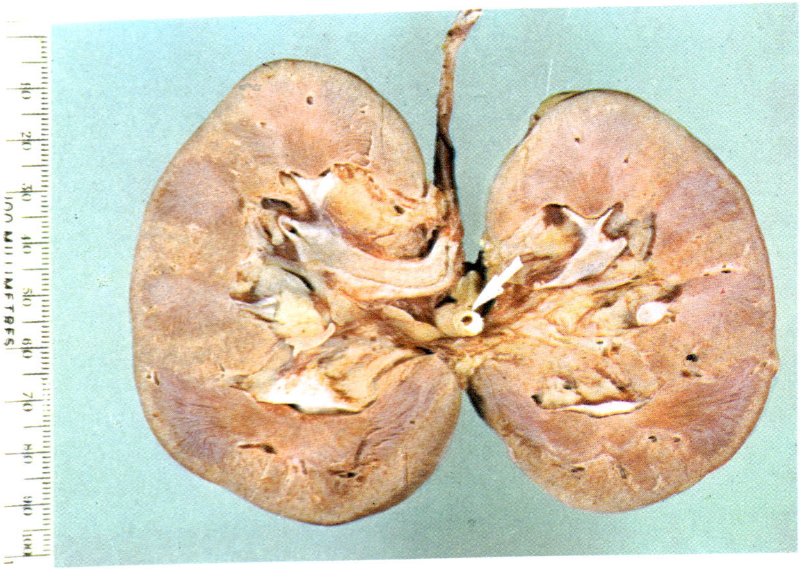

19

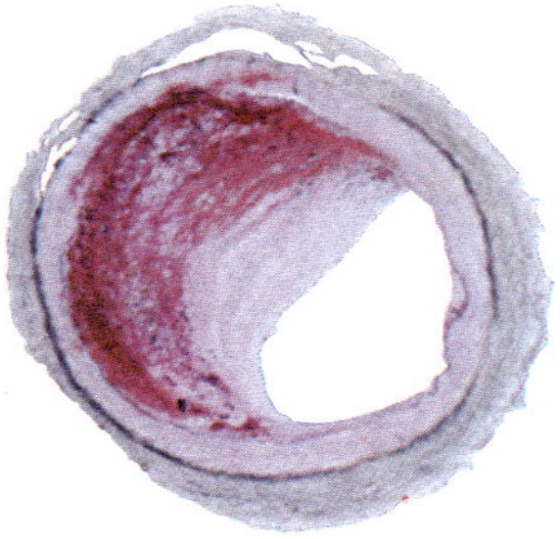

191 Gross pathology of renal artery stenosis (atherosclerotic).

192 Histology of renal artery stenosis due to atherosclerosis.

193, 194 Fibrous dysplasia (intimal) as a cause of renal artery stenosis in a young patient. There is a normal left and delayed right nephrogram (**193**), and the corresponding urogram demonstrates a small right kidney and constant filling defects in the upper ureter (arrows) due to notching by arterial collaterals (**194**).

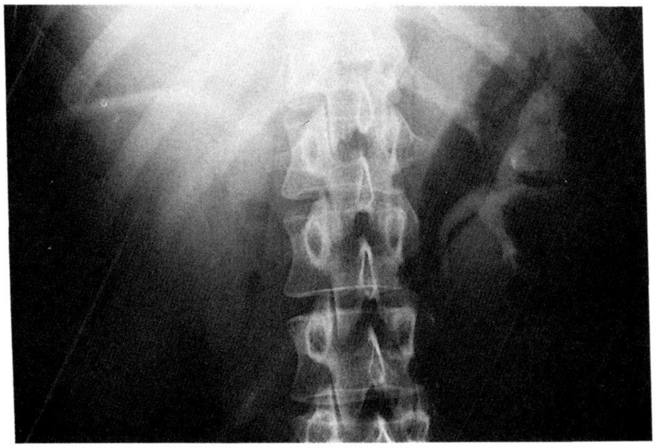

193

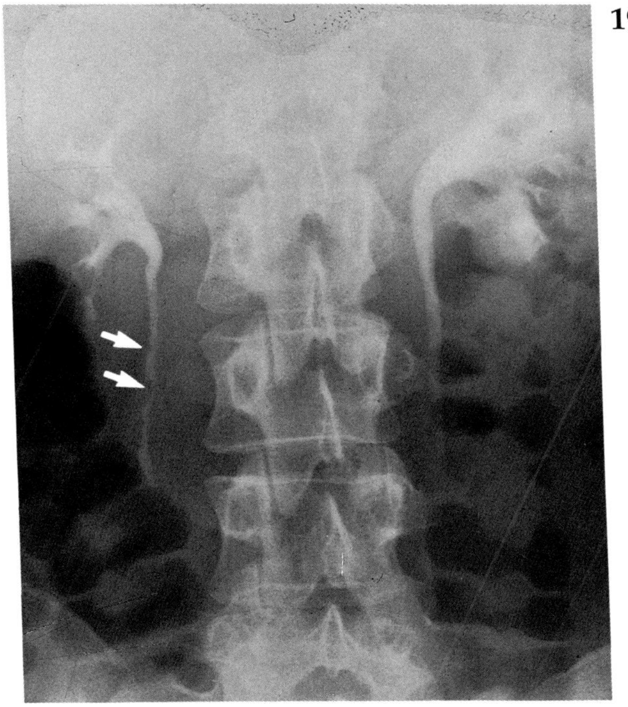

194

195

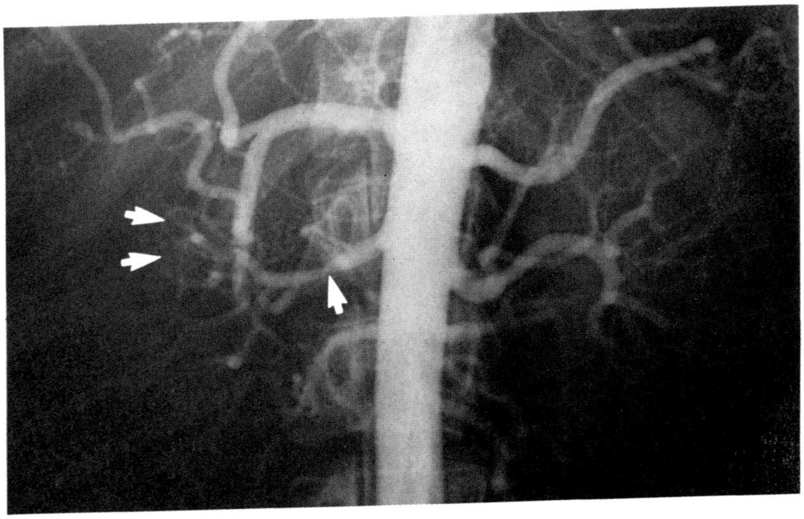

195–197 Flush aortogram of the patient in **193, 194,** demonstrating the collaterals (**195,** large arrows) formed in response to renal artery stenosis (small arrow). Selective right renal angiogram showing a smooth stenosis before (**196**, arrow), and after (**197**) balloon dilatation.

196

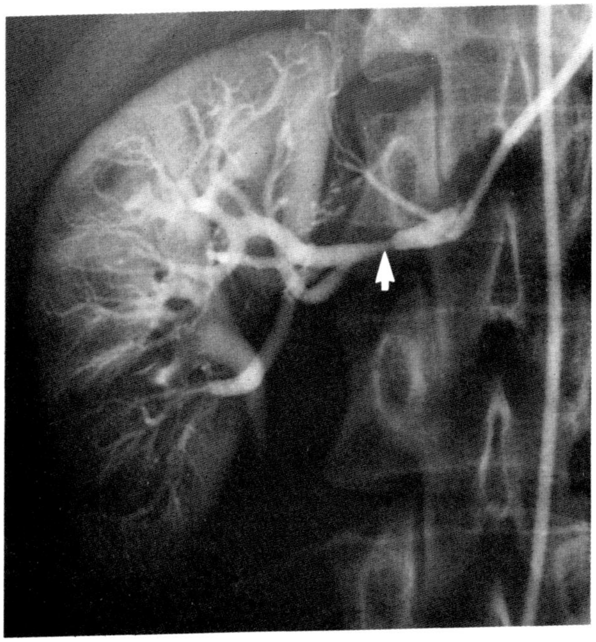

197

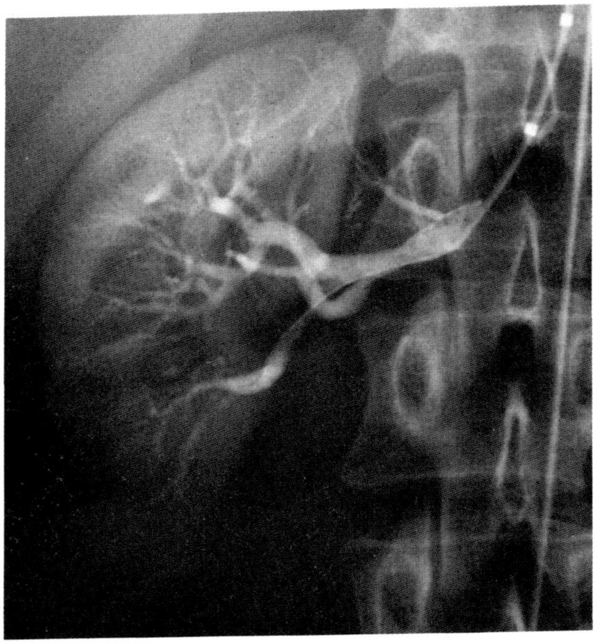

198

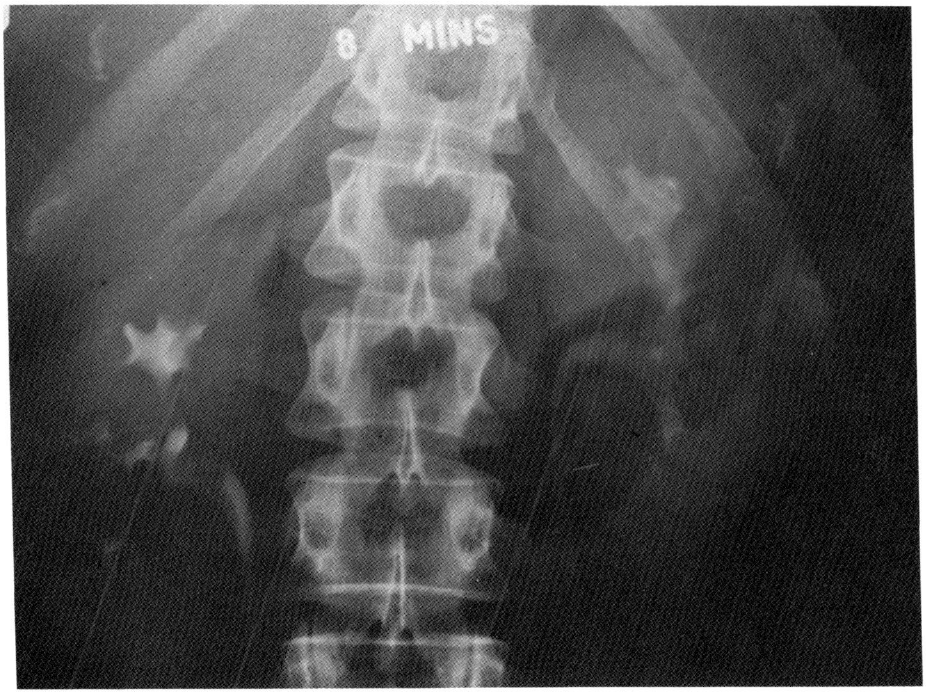

199

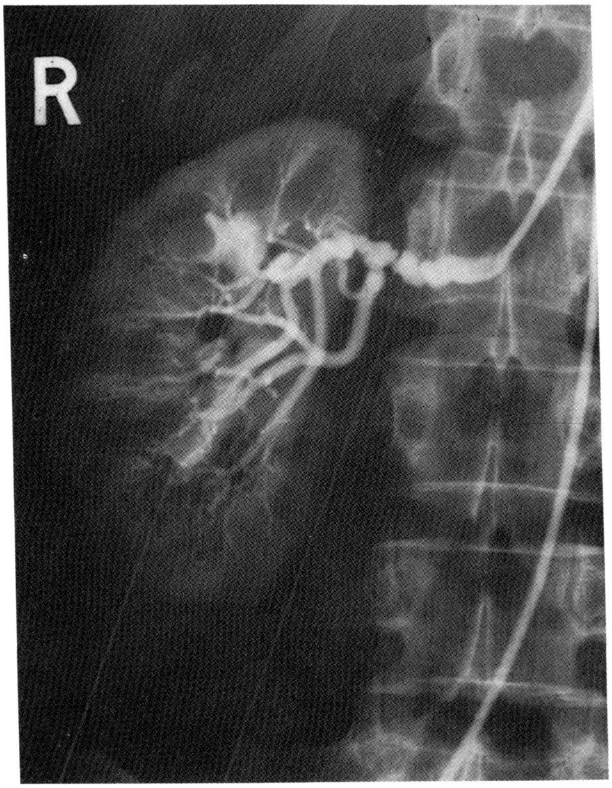

200

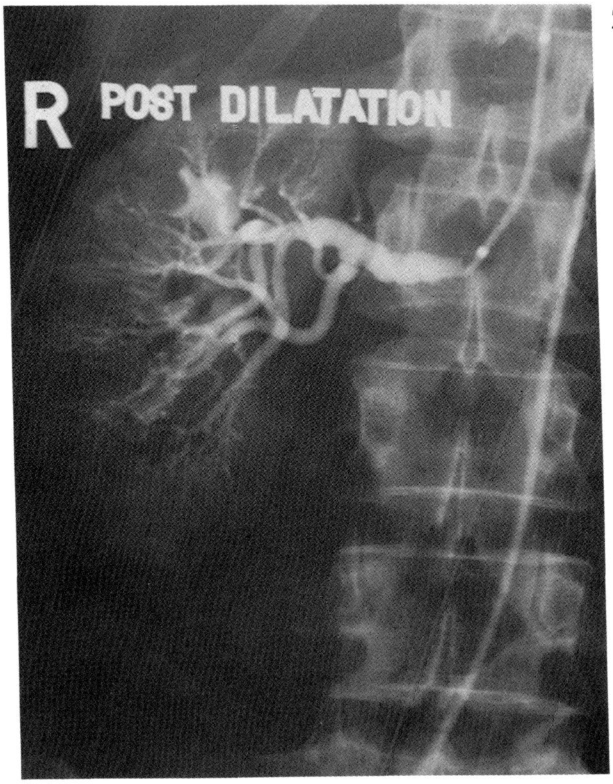

198–200 Fibromuscular renal artery stenosis. Due to reduced blood flow in the affected kidney, there is hyperconcentration of the excreted contrast medium causing a dense pyelogram in a small right kidney (**198**). The selective renal angiogram shows a beaded appearance with multiple stenoses (arrows) before (**199**) and after (**200**) balloon dilatation.

201

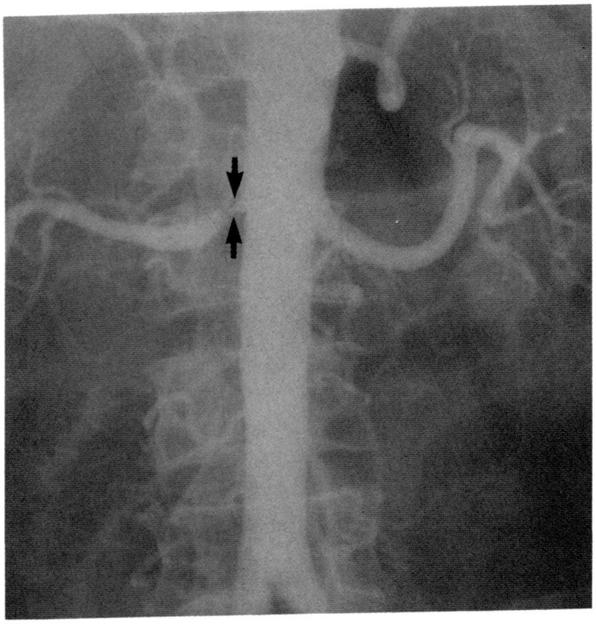

202

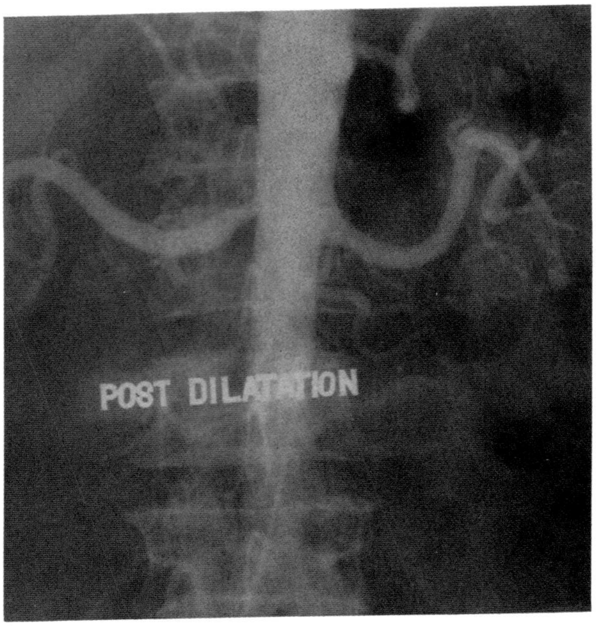

201, 202 Atherosclerotic renal artery stenosis in an elderly patient with other evidence of vascular disease. The flush aortogram shows a stenosis in the proximal renal artery (arrow, **201**) which undergoes balloon dilatation (**202**).

203

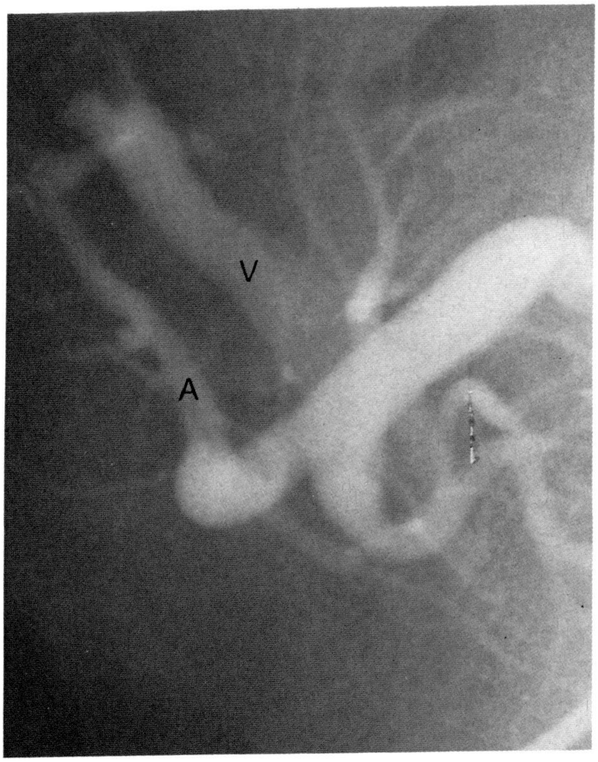

204

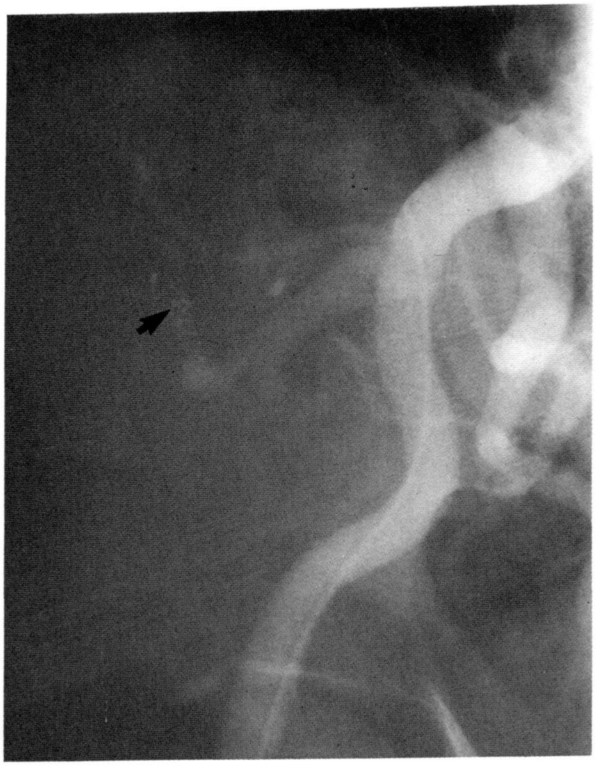

203, 204 Renal arteriovenous fistulae may be an occasional cause of hypertension. In this example an arteriovenous fistula (A: artery, V: vein) in a transplanted kidney is seen before (**203**) and after embolization with steel coils (**204**, arrow).

Coarctation of the aorta

Aortic coarctation is a congenital anomaly in which there is narrowing of the upper portion of the descending aorta at the site of the arterial duct. This accounts for approximately 5–8% of congenital heart disease, and as an isolated defect is more common in males than females.

Coarctation is frequently associated with other congenital heart disease. It may be associated with other anomalies, including Turner's, Noonan's, and congenital rubella syndromes. The most common extracardiac anomaly is an aneurysm of the Circle of Willis. In addition, it may be associated with a bicuspid aortic valve.

Coarctation of the aorta is a rare cause of hypertension which may be diagnosed by the physical findings. While adults present with hypertension and cardiovascular manifestations of the coarctation, in children the presentation may be with heart failure. The majority of patients with coarctation of the aorta are asymptomatic, although rarely, headache, cold extremities and claudication may be presenting features. Examination reveals markedly diminished or delayed femoral pulses with reduced or unobtainable systolic pressure in the legs and hypertension in the arms. Systolic and continuous murmurs over the lateral thoracic wall and scapulae may reflect dilated and tortuous collateral vessels. It is occasionally possible to hear a murmur over the anterior chest, back and spine directly from the coarctation. The chest radiograph often shows an abnormal aortic knuckle and rib notching. The diagnosis can be confirmed by echocardiography in younger patients, or by magnetic resonance imaging or angiography in older patients.

205

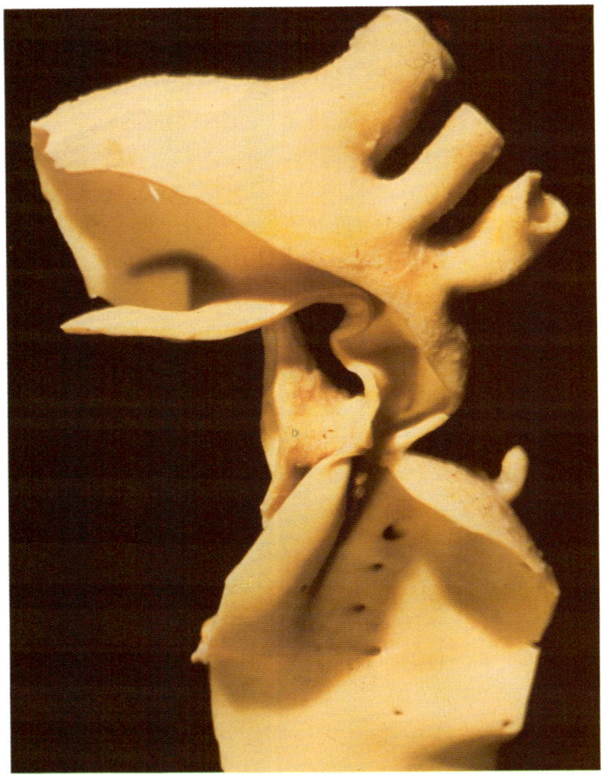

206

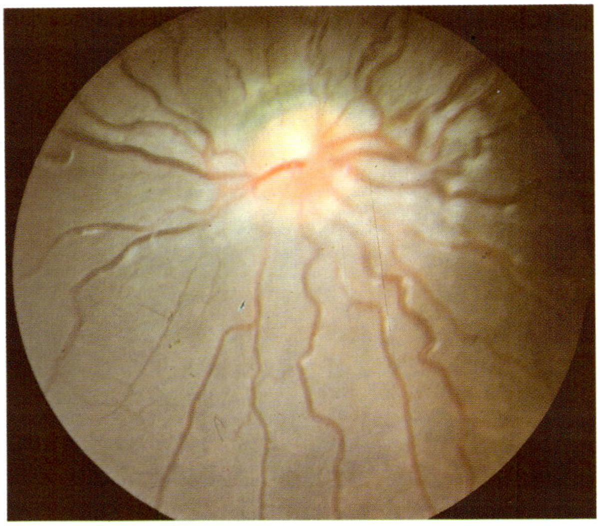

206 Retinal photograph in coarctation of the aorta showing tortuous vessels.

205 Pathology of coarctation of the aorta showing a discrete shelf-like narrowing of the aorta below the left subclavian artery. In this case there is dilatation of the arch of the aorta and the area immediately following the stenosis.

207

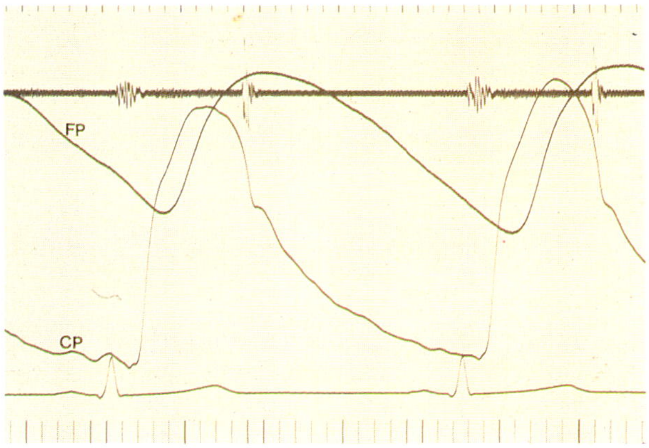

207 Physical signs in coarction of the aorta. While the carotid pulse (CP) is normal, there is delay and prolongation of the femoral pulse (FP) recorded by indirect pulse transducers.

208

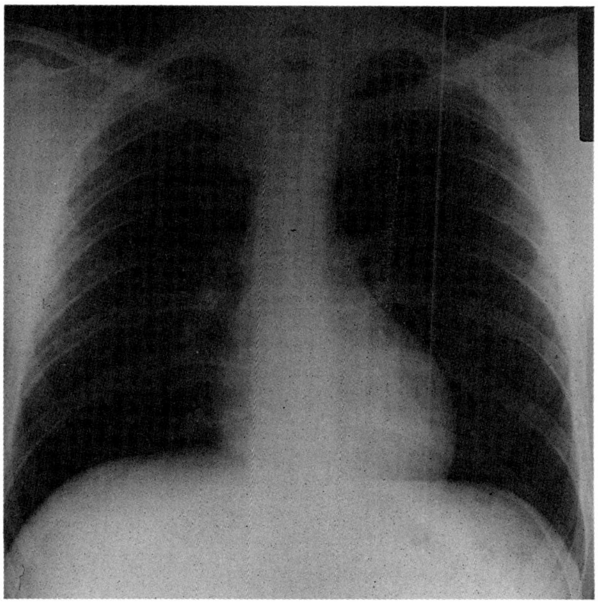

209

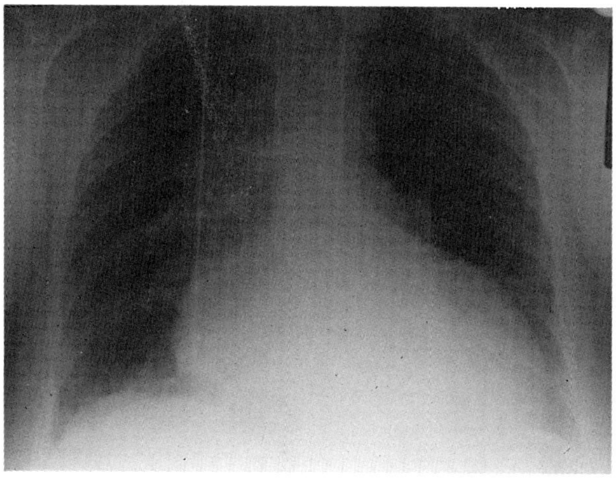

210

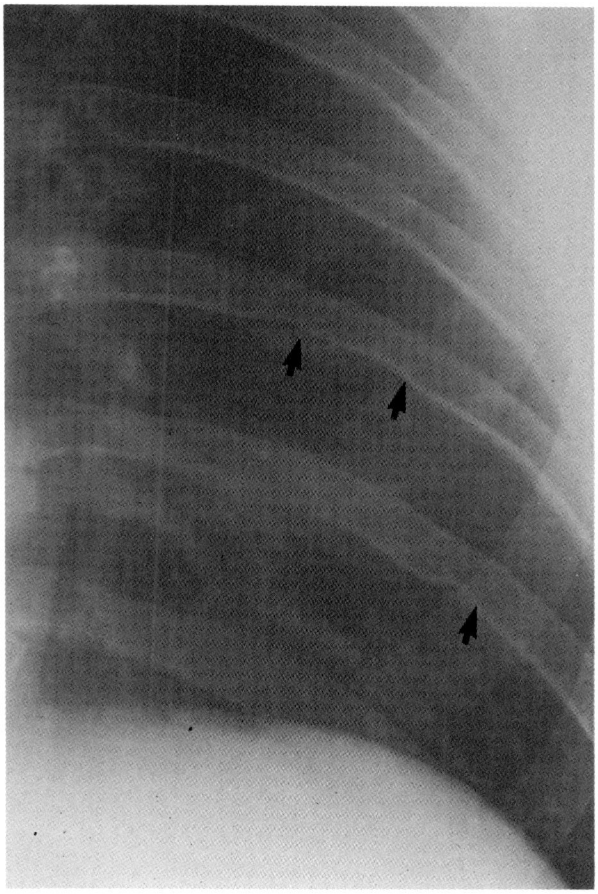

208–210 Chest radiographs with both a small (**208**), and a large heart (**209**), in patients with coarctation of the aorta. In both, an abnormal aortic knuckle and rib notching are seen. The rib notching (arrows) is shown more clearly in a magnified view (**210**).

211

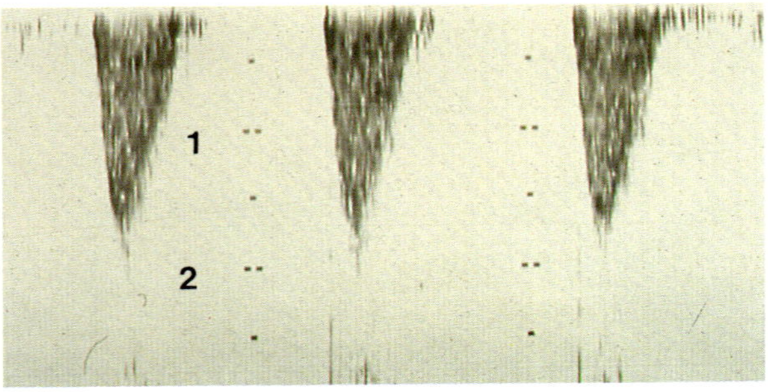

21

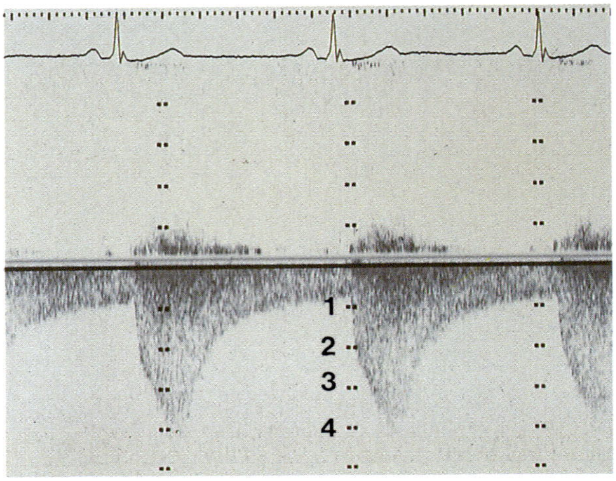

211, 212 Continuous-wave Doppler recordings taken from the supersternal notch showing an increased velocity of blood away from the transducer across the stenosis of the coarctation. **211** shows a mild coarctation with a velocity of almost 2 m per second, representing a gradient of less than 16 mmHg in a post-operative stenosis. **212**, however, presents a severe coarctation of the aorta with a peak velocity of 4 m per second (gradient of 64 mmHg). In addition, there is a continuous velocity trace across the obstruction representing continuing flow throughout diastole.

213

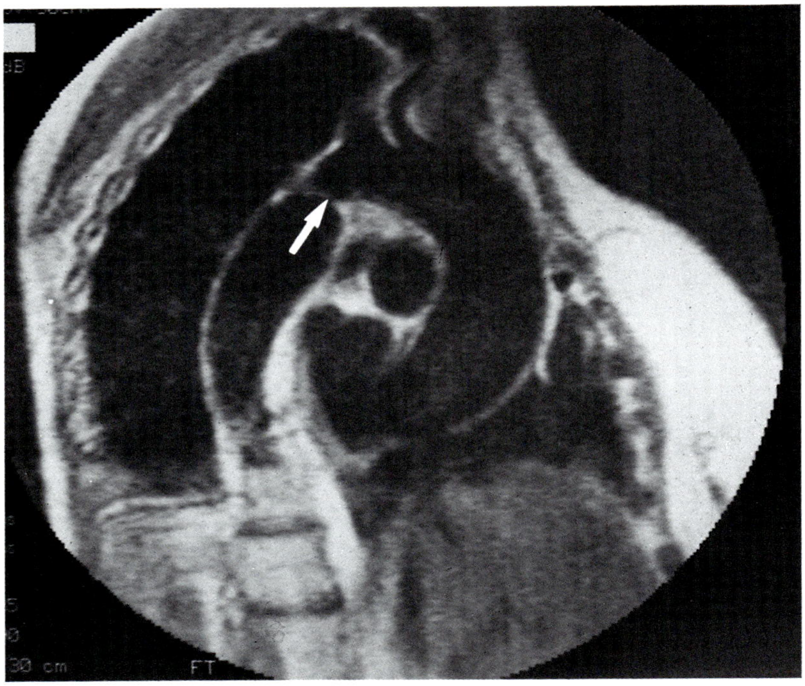

21

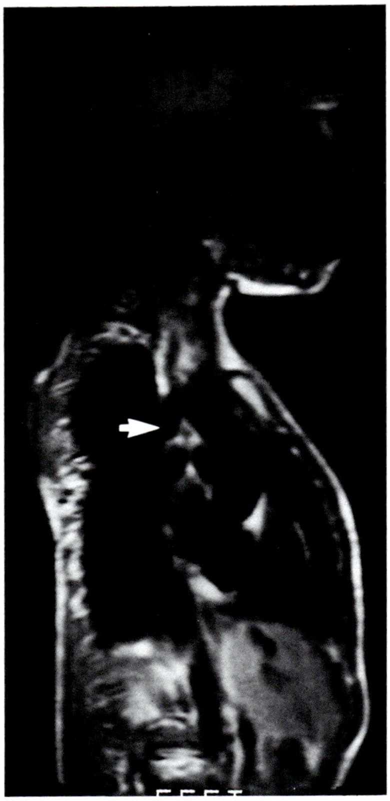

213, 214 Magnetic resonance scans: sagittal sections in coarctation of the aorta. **213** shows a dilated ascending aorta with a diaphragmatic obstruction in the first part of the descending aorta (arrow). **214** demonstrates restenosis of a coarctation following an end-to-end surgical repair (arrow). There was a persistent gradient across this area of stenosis with resultant hypertension. This restenosis was treated by percutaneous balloon dilatation.

215

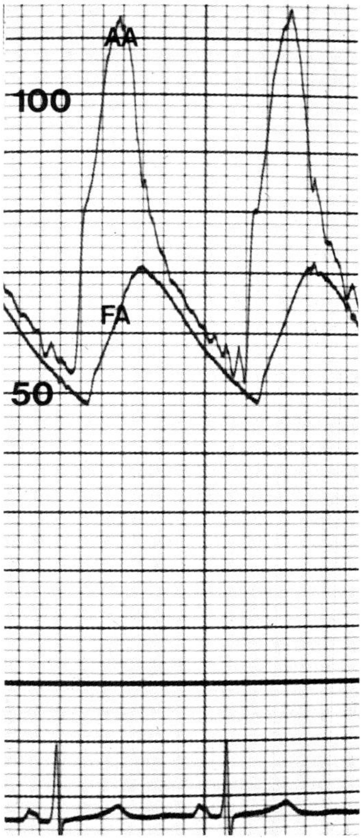

215 Pressure trace in coarctation of the aorta showing a large volume pulse in the ascending aorta (AA) and a smaller volume, lower pressure pulse in the femoral artery (FA).

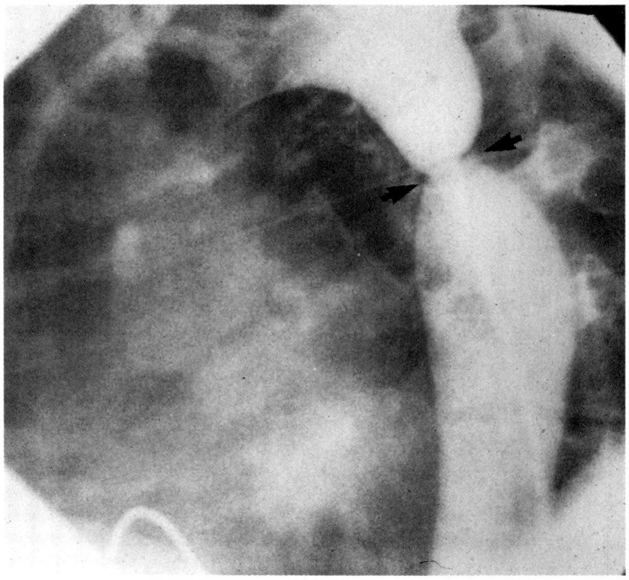

216

216 Left anterior oblique projection of the ascending aortogram in a patient with coarctation of the aorta. This shows a discrete eccentric narrowing just below the left subclavian artery (arrows).

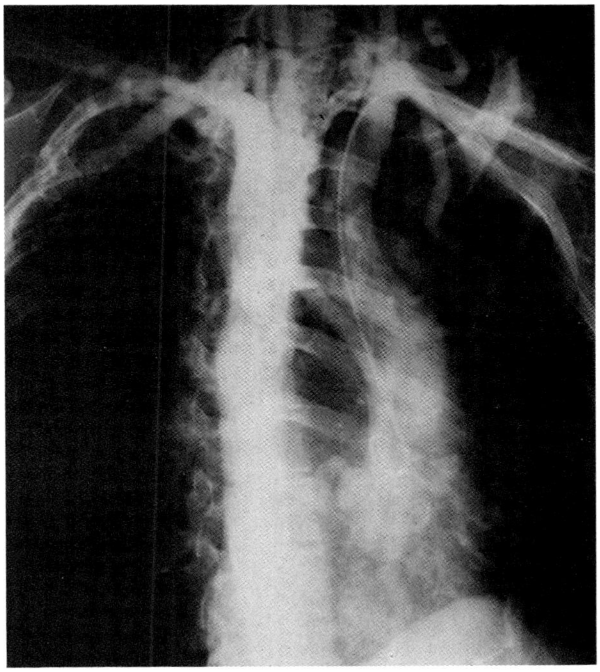

217

217 Aortogram in a coarctation showing collateral vessels.

218

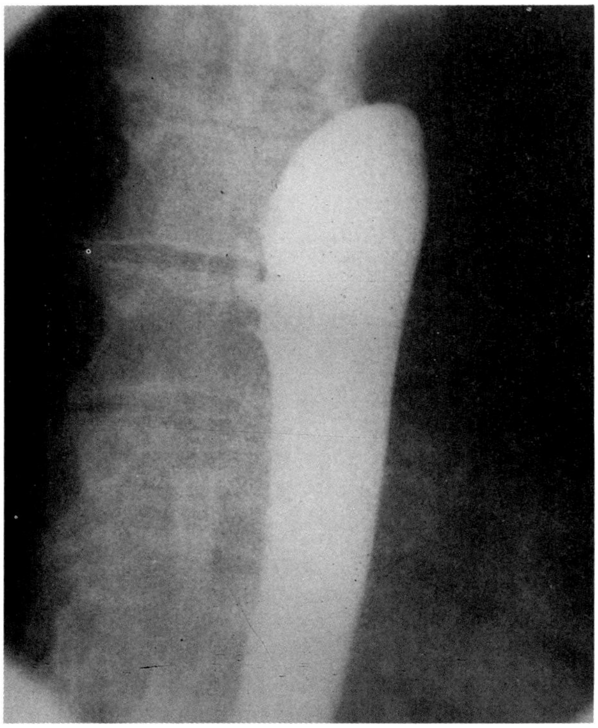

218 Occasionally the coarctation leads to complete interruption of the aorta in the region of the coarctation. This is shown here on a descending aortogram.

219

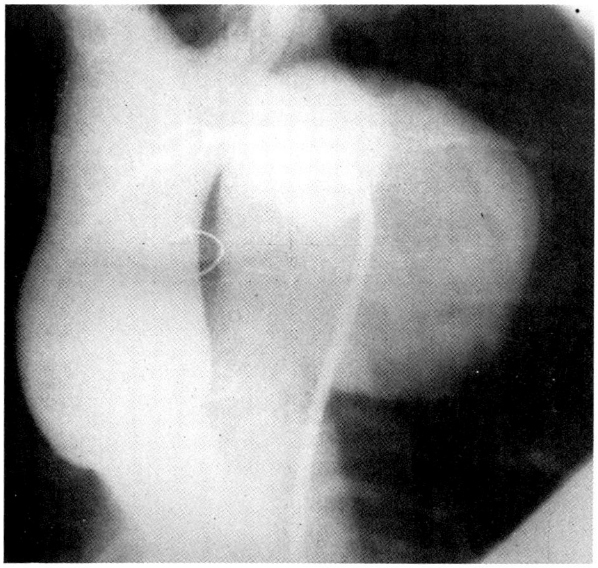

219 Following repair or dilatation of the coarctation of the aorta, hypertension may persist through unknown central and baroreceptor mechanisms. Despite relief of the stenosis in the area of coarctation, aneurysms may develop, as shown in this figure. There is no apparent connection between aneurysm formation and persistent hypertension.

220

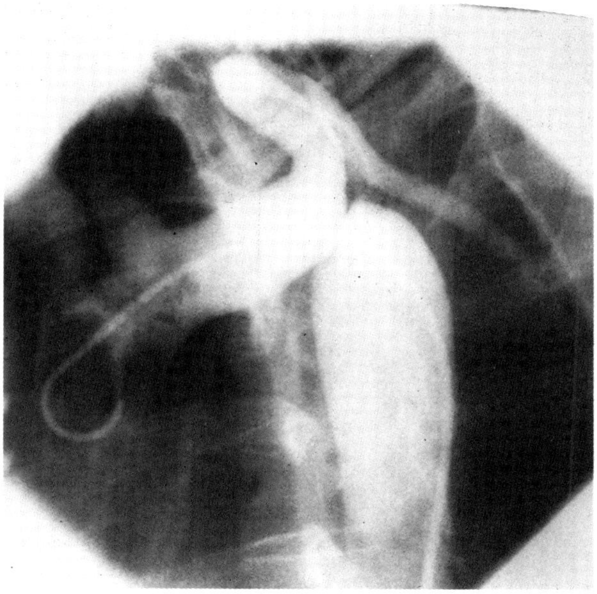

221

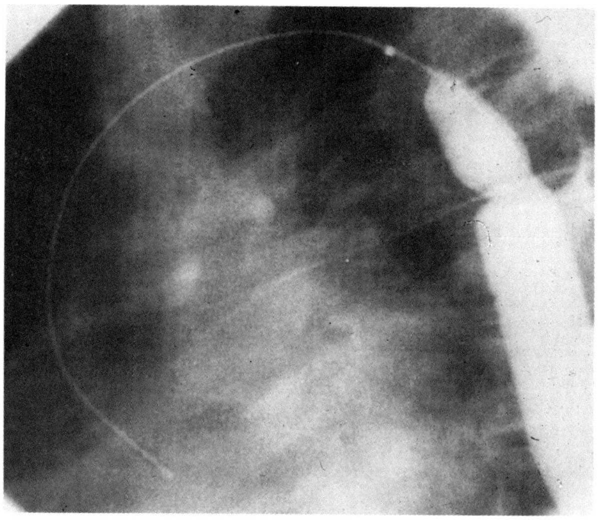

222

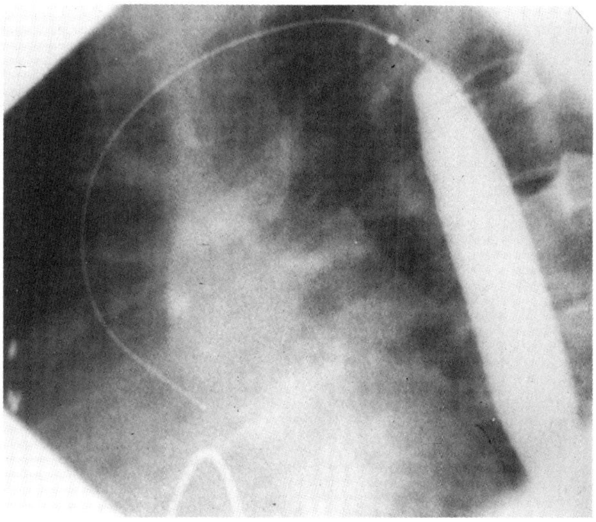

223

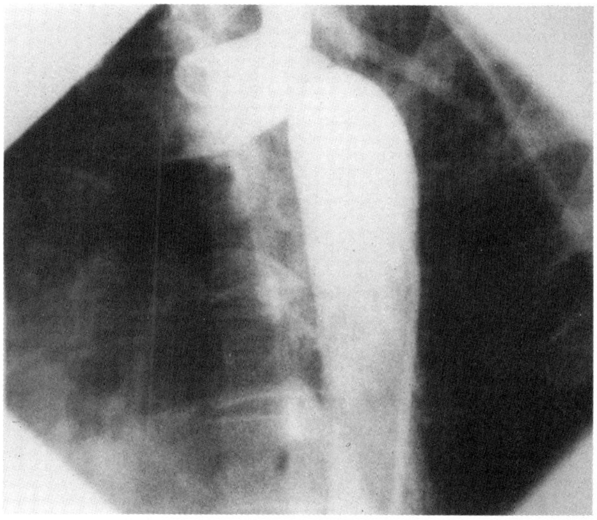

220–223 Left anterior oblique projection showing a coarctation (**220**). A balloon is inflated partially (**221**) and then fully (**222**) across the stenosis. This relieves the obstruction both haemodynamically and angiographically (**223**). The technique of balloon dilatation is most useful in post-operative restenosis but may also be used in native coarctations as shown here.

Takayasu's arteritis

This uncommon form of large vessel arteritis is rarely seen in the west. It is much more common in women, and in three-quarters of patients hypertension is one of the presenting features. Hypertension appears to arise through several mechanisms, including acquired coarctation and renal artery stenosis.

224

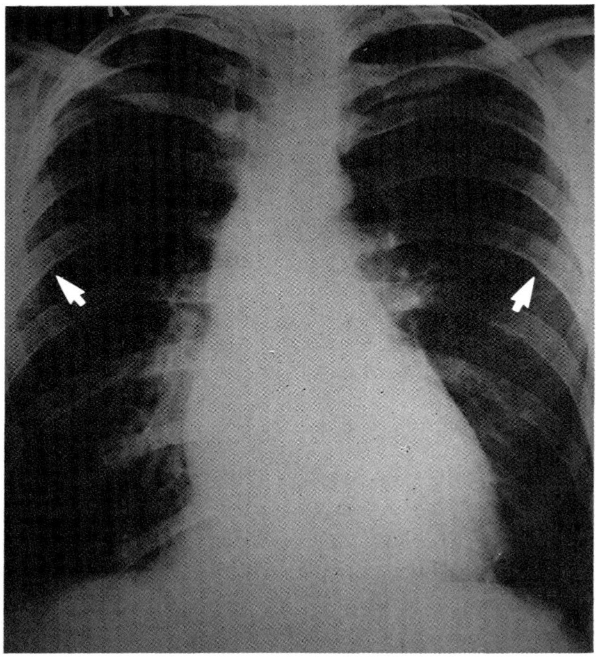

224 Chest radiograph showing mild cardiomegaly with rib notching (arrows) from acquired coarctation in Takayasu's arteritis.

225

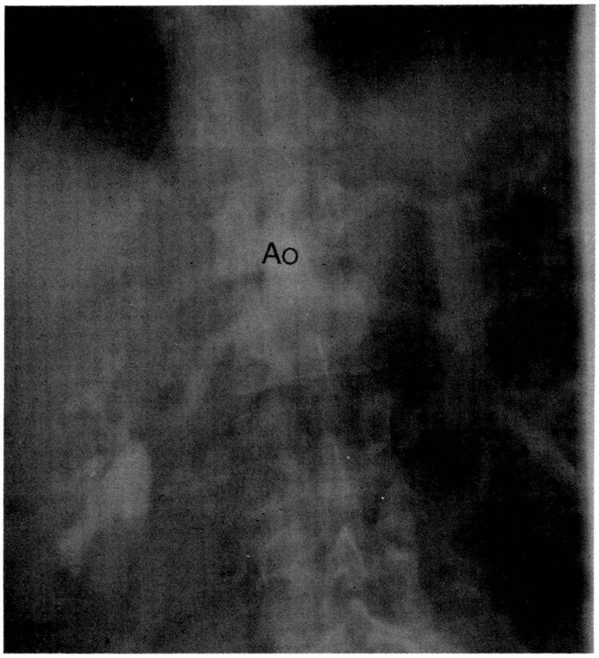

225 Arch aortogram showing an aortic obstruction in the case of 224. Filling of only a small part of the descending aorta (Ao) in the region of the renal arteries is seen.

Effects of hypertension

Vital to the assessment of the hypertensive patient is the identification of target organ damage. This may be seen in the retina, the arterial tree, the left ventricle and the kidney.

The degree of target organ damage may vary considerably from patient to patient for the same level of blood pressure elevation. Vascular damage can best be determined by examination of the fundus, heart and kidney.

Effects of hypertension on the eye

In 1939 Keith, Wegener and Barker described fundal vascular changes in both hypertensive and atherosclerotic patients. The retinopathy in both groups of patients may be graded as:

- Grade I — narrowing of the arteriolar lumen;
- Grade II — sclerosis of the adventitia and thickening of the arteriolar wall, visible as arteriovenous nipping.

In hypertensive patients, two further grades are recognized:

- Grade III—rupture of small vessels occuring with progressive hypertension, and seen as haemorrhages and exudates.
- Grade IV—This grade of hypertensive retinopathy also includes papilloedema.

The majority of these patients are asymptomatic, though there may be visual loss in grade III and grade IV hypertensive retinopathy. The presence of these higher degrees of retinopathy is associated with a greatly elevated risk of subsequent mortality and morbidity.

226

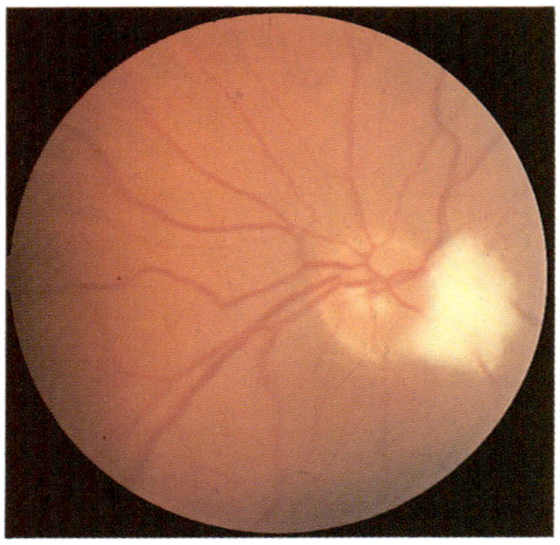

226 Normal optic fundus. There are medullated fibres seen in this normal fundus.

227

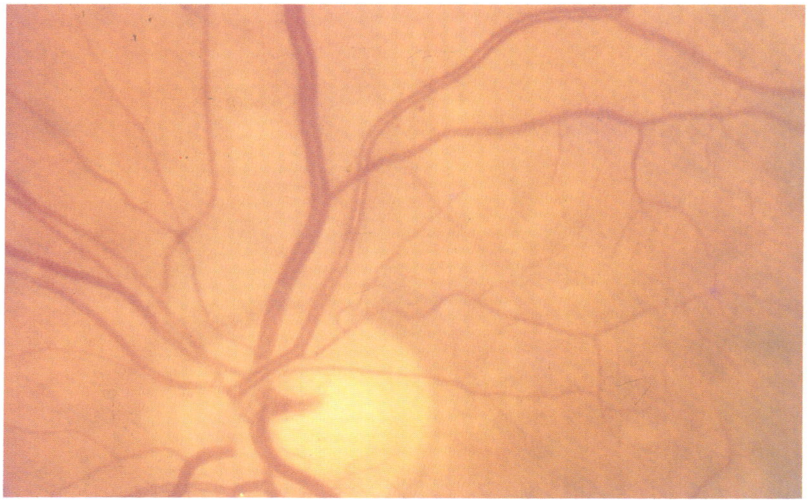

227 Grade I hypertensive retinopathy. The changes seen in this optic fundus include silver wiring of the arteries.

228

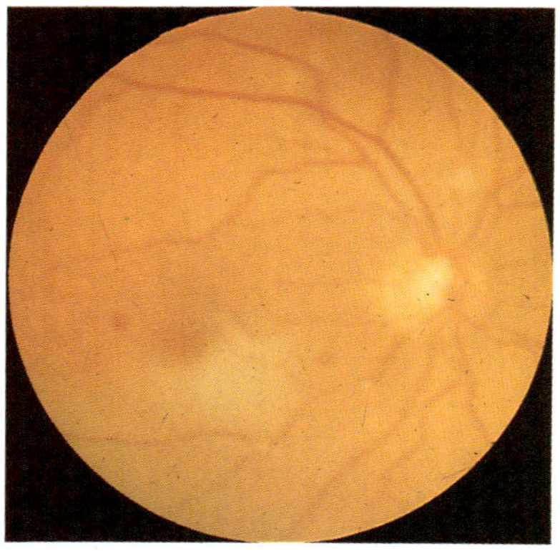

228 Grade II hypertensive retinopathy with haemorrhages and exudates.

229 Grade III hypertensive retinopathy with extensive areas of flame-shaped haemorrhages.

229

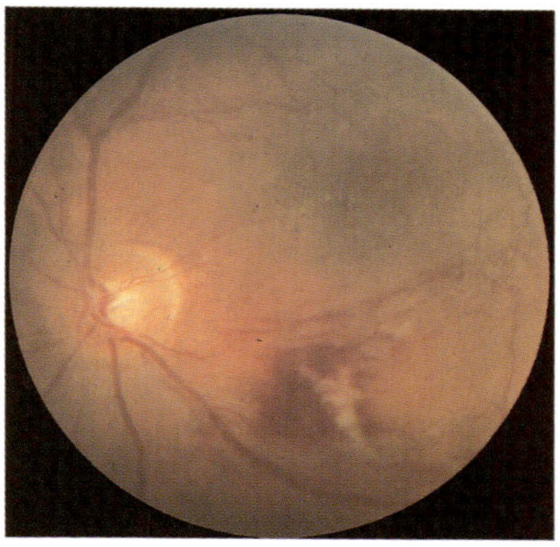

230

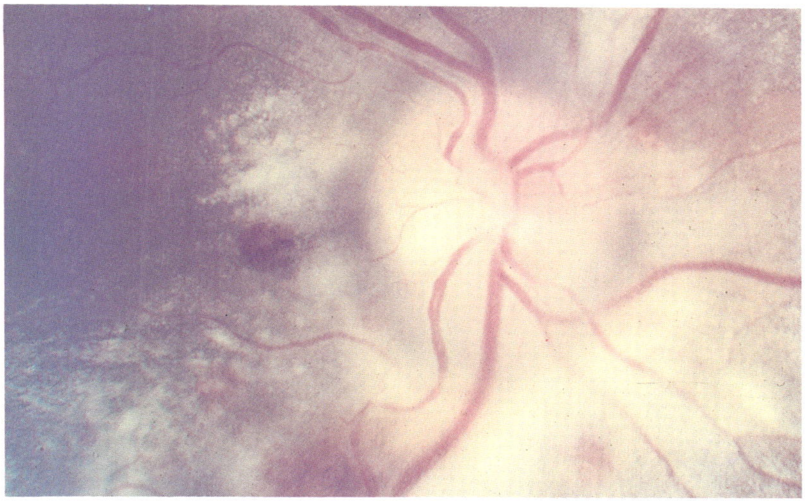

230 Grade IV hypertensive retinopathy showing papilloedema and small areas of haemorrhage.

231 Severe grade IV hypertensive retinopathy showing papilloedema and large haemorrhages.

231

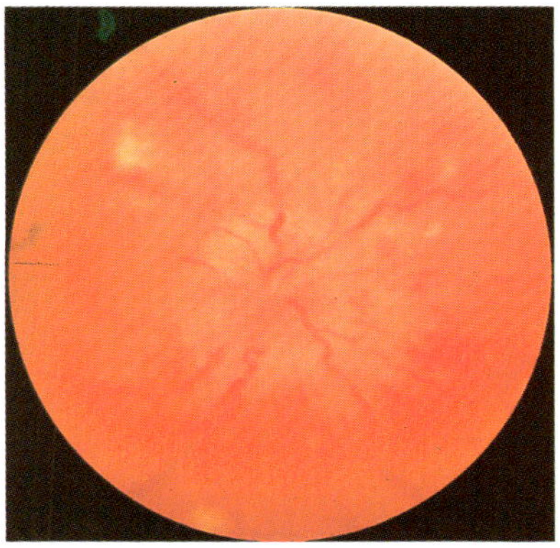

Effects of hypertension on the kidney

The severity of hypertension is often reflected by morphological changes in the kidney. In primary or essential hypertension, morphological abnormalities occur subsequent to a period of raised blood pressure. Alternatively, in secondary renal hypertension, raised blood pressure is a consequence of an established renal abnormality. In secondary hypertension from other causes, changes in the kidney in general are similar to those of essential hypertension.

Abnormalities are basically those of 'age changes', i.e. vascular sclerosis and ischaemia, but are more severe than expected for the age of the patient. Benign nephrosclerosis is the term used for the renal changes of benign hypertension (**234, 235**).

232

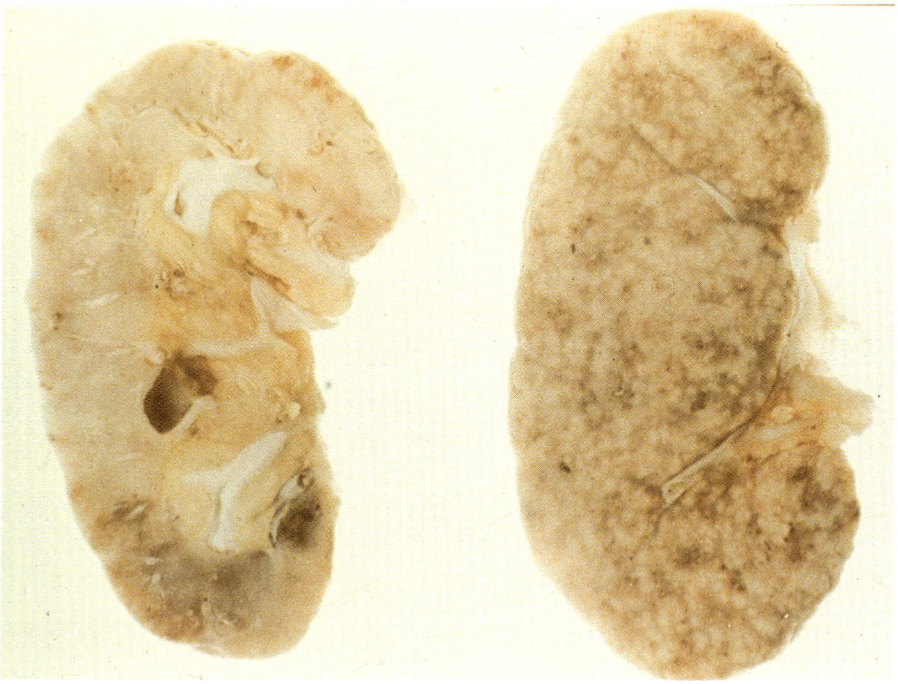

232 The kidneys may be normal or moderately reduced in size. The cortical surfaces have a fine granularity due to the alteration of the normal or hypertrophic parenchyma with foci of ischaemic scarring. As the renal abnormalities progress, there is cortical narrowing and thickening of the intrarenal arteries.

233 Small arteries show medial hypertrophy and widening of the intima secondary to concentric fibroelastic proliferation. Onion skinning is a typical histological finding. Such abnormalities are present to some degree in normal individuals over the age of 50 years, but are more severe and occur at a younger age in hypertension (EPS × 200).

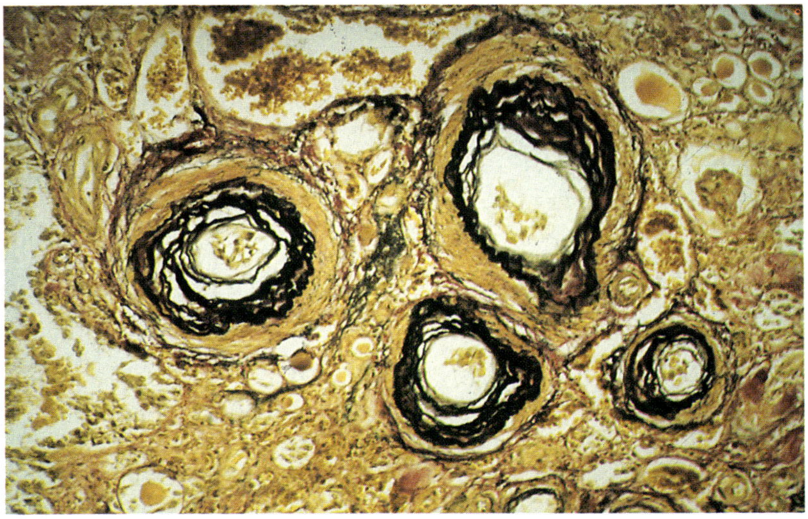

233

234 Renal histology showing arteriolar sclerosis. There is extreme hypo/acellular eosinophilic thickening of the wall with loss of muscle cells of the media (H & E × 400).

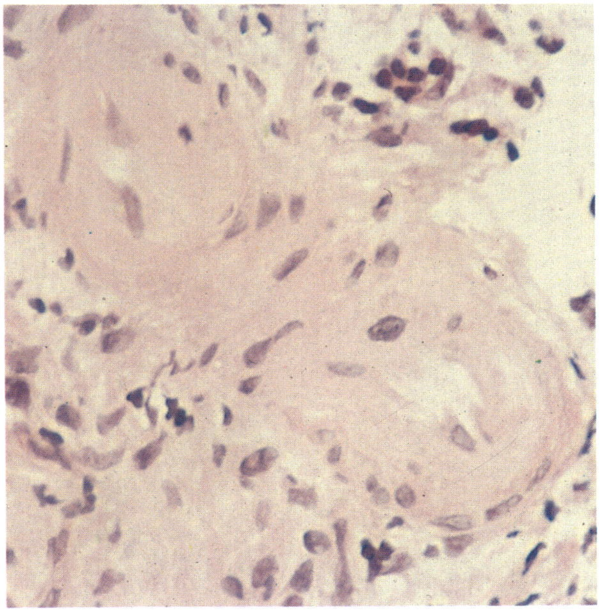

234

235 Renal histology showing prominent juxta-glomerular apparatus (JGA). There is an increase in the cells of the JGA at the glomerular hilum. Note that these cells are confined to the area between the hilum and the distal tubule, which is lined by small dark cells (PAS × 400).

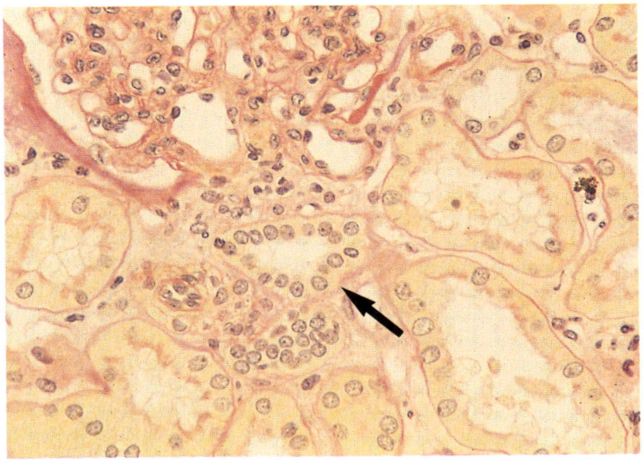

235

236 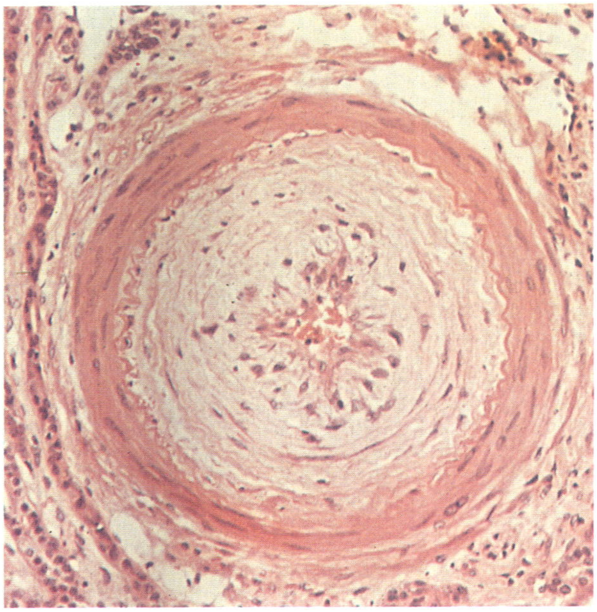

The following changes are seen in malignant hypertension (**236–240**).

236 Small artery showing extreme luminal narrowing secondary to concentric myointimal cellular proliferation. The wall has a blue–grey tinge and a mucoid appearance that is indicative of active proliferation. This type of concentric onion-skin appearance is typical of severe hypertension (H & E × 400).

237 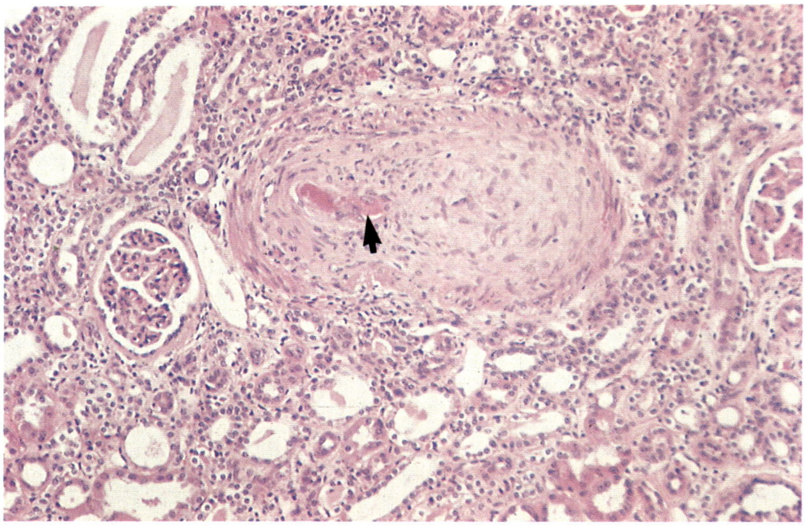

237 Lower power view of the same section as **236**. Another vessel with essentially similar changes but with super-added fibrin thrombus occluding the lumen (arrow). Note the surrounding renal parenchyma showing ischaemic changes of glomerular shrinkage and tubular atrophy (H & E × 100).

238 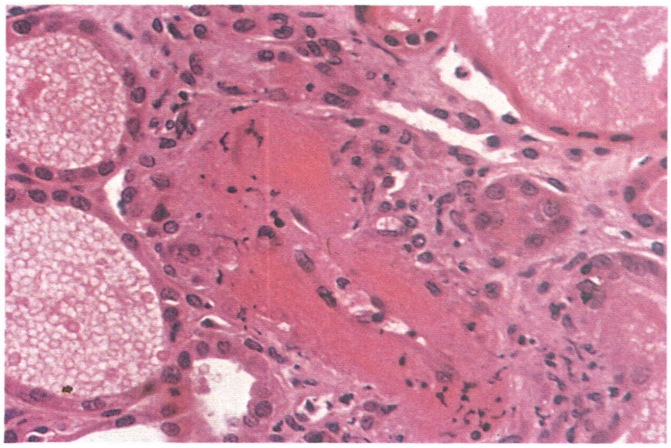

238 Fibrinoid necrosis of an arteriole (H & E × 400).

239 Arteriole at a glomerular hilum (G) showing myo-intimal onion skin proliferation, severely narrowed lumen, and focal fibrinoid necrosis of the wall (stained red, arrow) (MSB × 400).

239

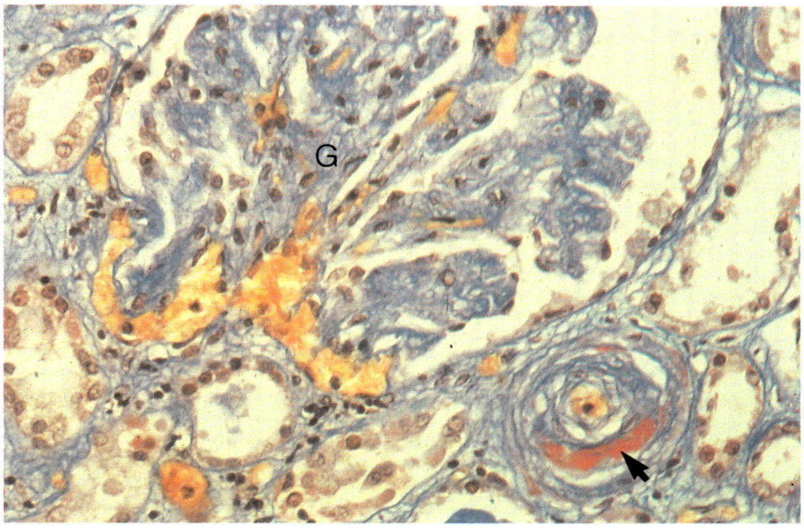

240 Severe hypertensive vascular changes similar to **238**. Sections are from a patient with end-stage glomerulonephritis and secondary renal hypertension. The vascular abnormalities are essentially similar to those in primary malignant hypertension. The viable glomeruli, however, have the stigmata of a proliferative glomerulonephritis. Tubular atrophy is marked (H & E × 100).

240

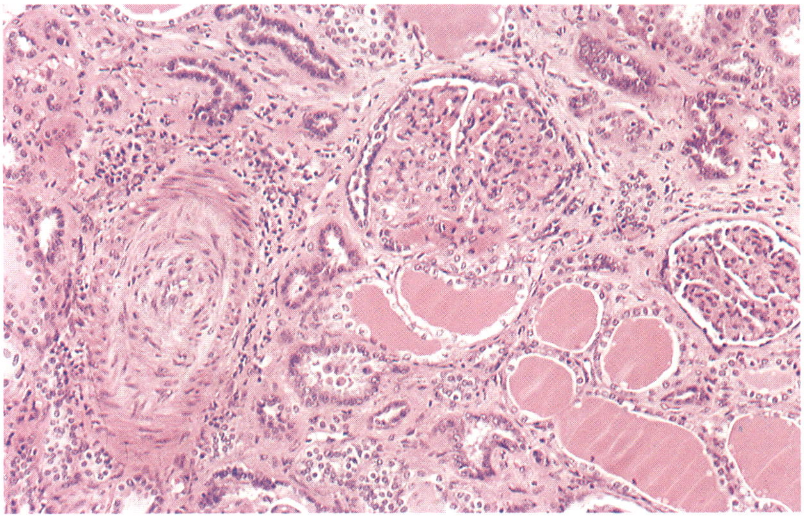

241 Renal angiogram in benign nephrosclerosis with a small irregular kidney. The investigation was performed to exclude renal artery stenosis.

241

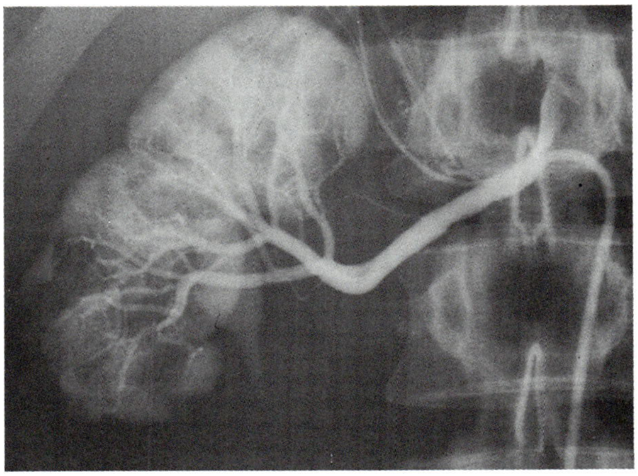

Left ventricular hypertrophy

One of the earliest responses to chronically elevated blood pressure is thickening of the left ventricular wall. It is important to identify hypertrophy, as it has now been identified as an independent risk factor for the development of coronary artery disease.

While the majority of patients with hypertensive left ventricular hypertrophy will be asymptomatic, a small proportion of these will develop breathlessness and angina in the absence of large coronary artery disease. This is due to impairment of relaxation and filling of the left ventricle. These abnormalities may become extreme in elderly women with only mildly elevated blood pressure. Such patients may have normal systolic function with gross ventricular hypertrophy and abnormalities of relaxation filling, leading to symptomatic heart failure.

242

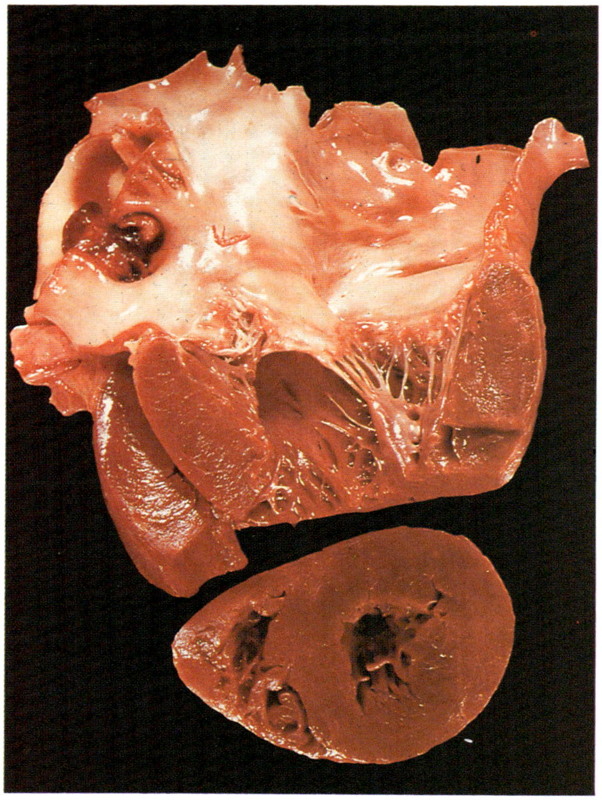

242 The heart has been opened to show severe concentric left ventricular hypertrophy due to long-standing systemic hypertension.

24.

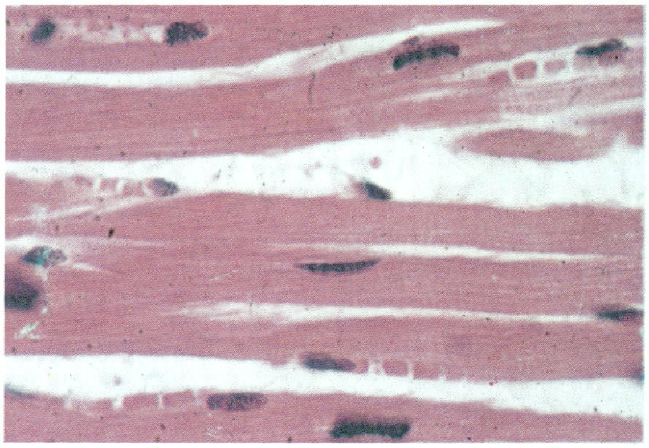

243 Histology of normal left ventricular myocardial fibres; compare with **244**.

24

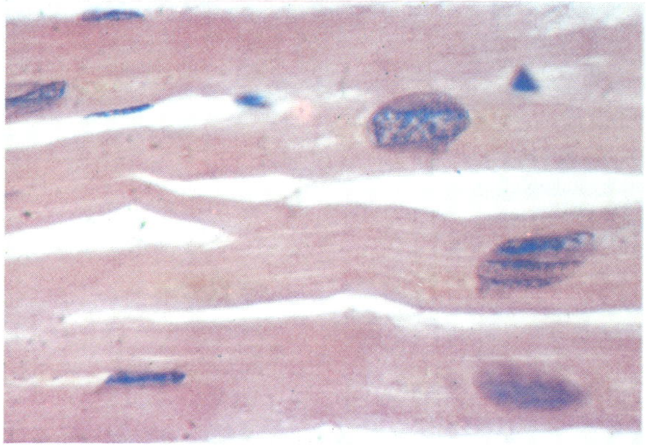

244 Hypertrophied left ventricular myocardial fibres. Note the difference in muscle fibre thickness, size and shape of nuclei.

245 Mild left ventricular hypertrophy has no physical findings, but as the degree of wall thickening and myocardial dysfunction becomes more severe, there could be the development of a fourth heart sound (phonocardiogram, S_4) and a prominent a-wave in the cardiac impulse (tall a-wave in the upstroke of the apexcardiogram).

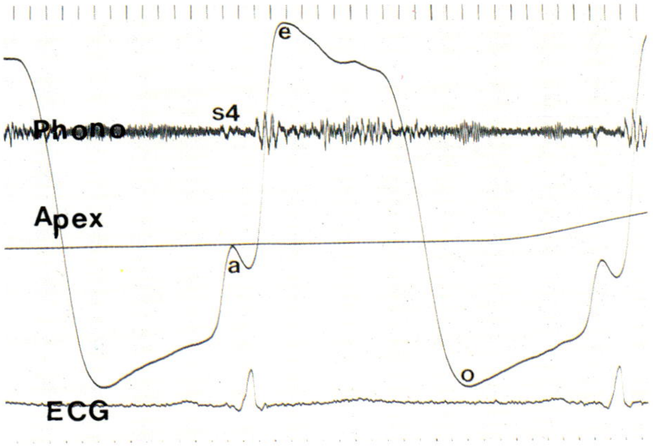

245

246

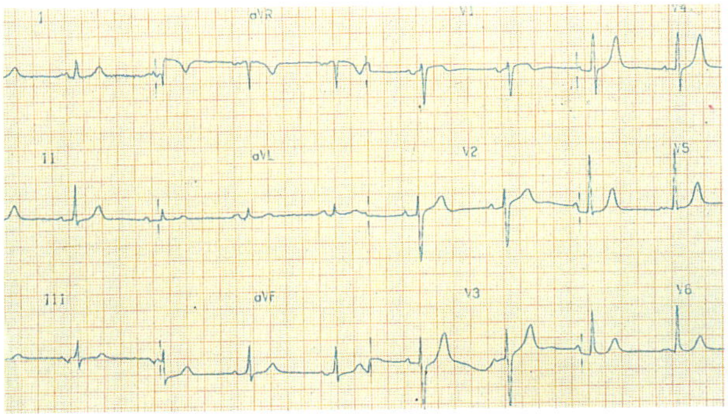

247

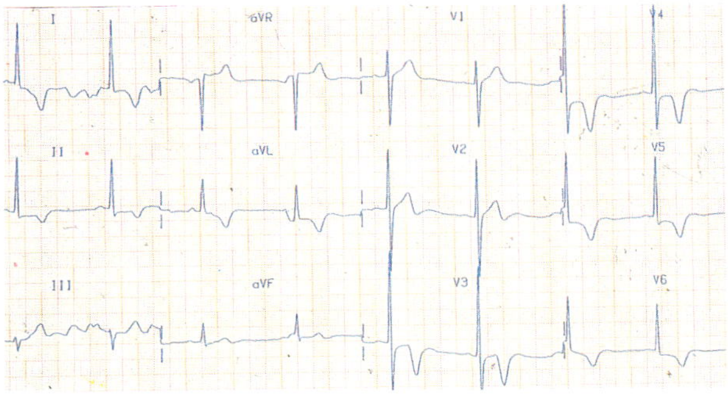

246 Electrocardiogram with left atrial enlargement as an expression of left ventricular hypertrophy without QRS voltage increase or ST segment changes. Left atrial enlargement is evidenced by bifasic P-waves in lead VI.

247 Electrocardiogram showing severe left ventricular hypertrophy with increased QRS voltage and marked ST segment depression with T-wave inversion in the lateral precordial leads.

248 Chest radiograph in a patient with severe hypertension. There is slight left ventricular predominance but otherwise the chest X-ray is within normal limits. Despite the presence of a normal chest radiograph, the echocardiogram confirms the presence of severe ventricular hypertrophy.

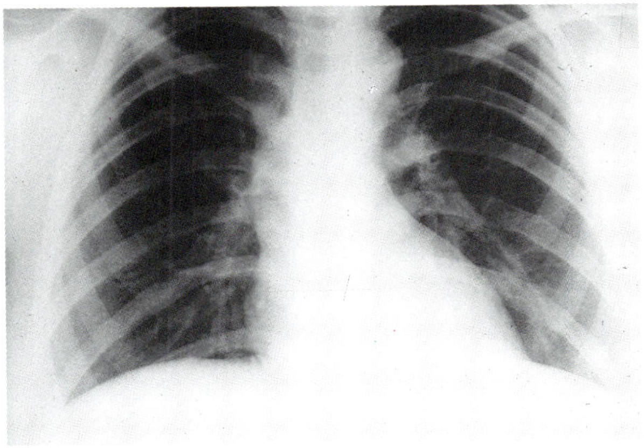

248

249

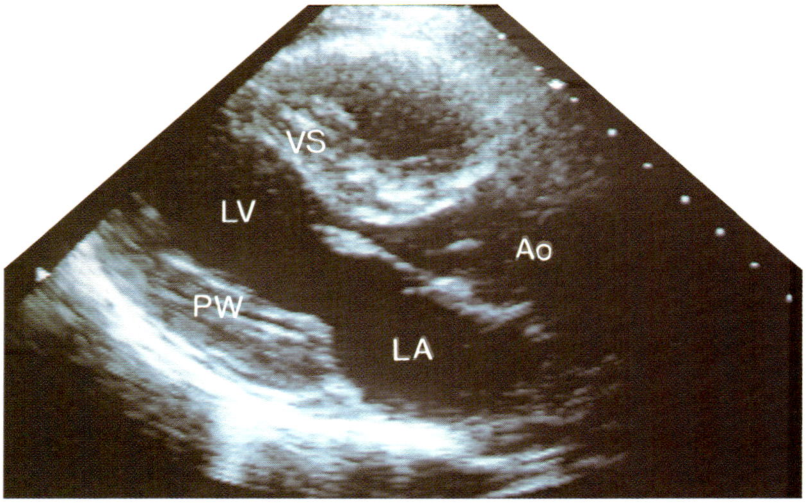

249–251 Echocardiograms in the parasternal long axis (**249** diastole, **250** systole), and short axis (**251**). There is moderate left ventricular hypertrophy with thickening of the interventricular septum (VS) and posterior wall (PW).

250

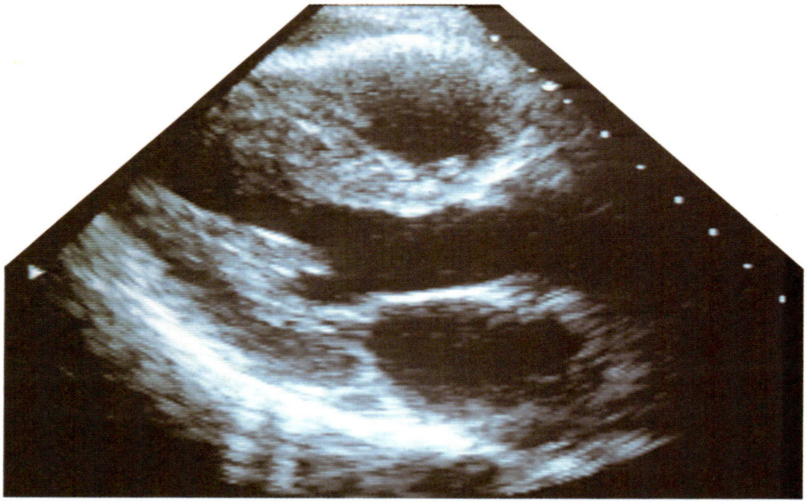

251

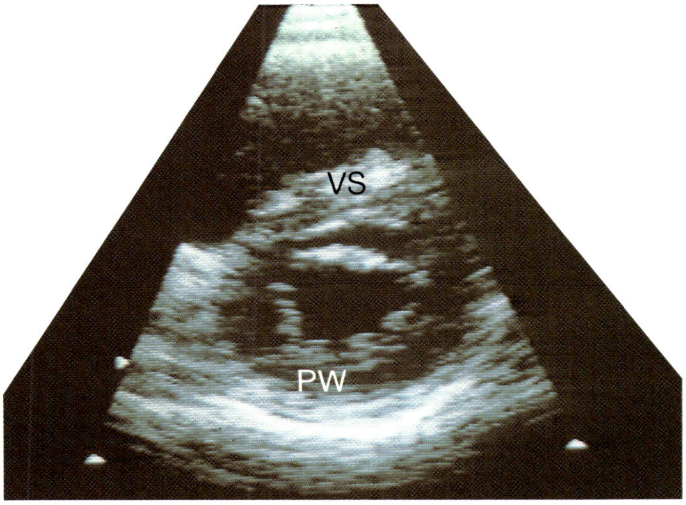

252 Abnormalities of diastolic left ventricular function may be demonstrated by a variety of techniques, including digitized M-mode echocardiography, gated blood pool scanning, and Doppler ultrasound. The latter is technically the most simple to perform. The mitral valve inflow shows a normal initial peak (E) but a very prominent a-wave (a). This is a reflection of abnormal diastolic left ventricular properties.

252

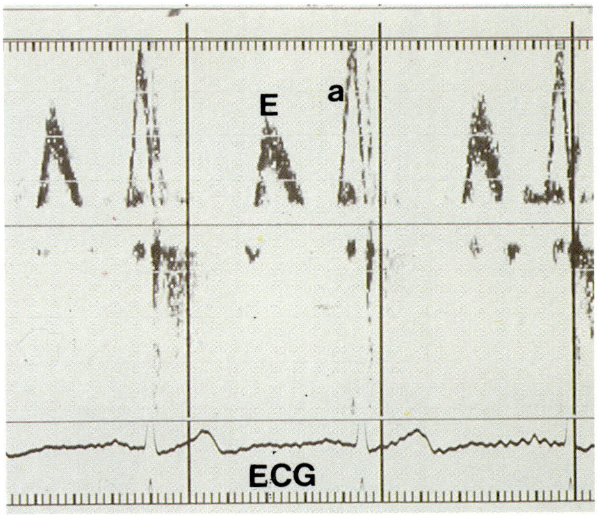

253

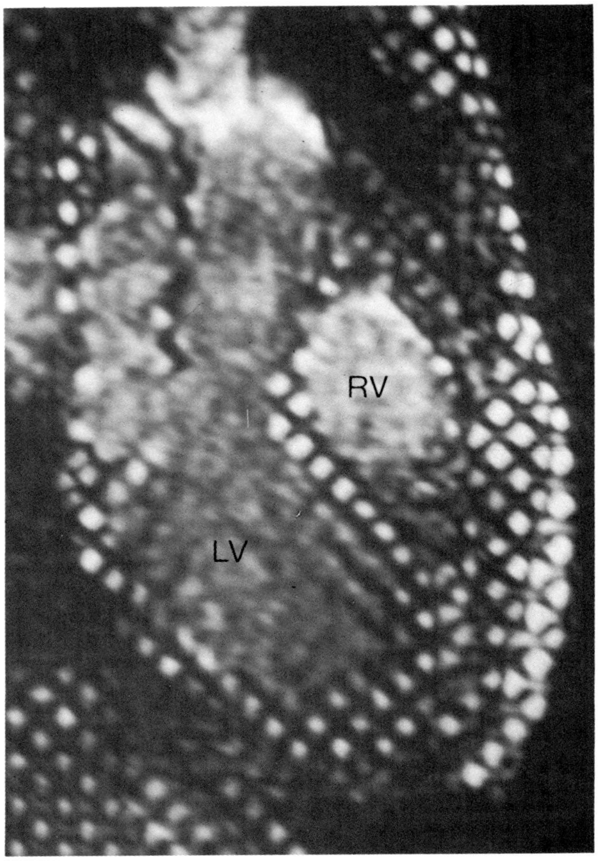

254

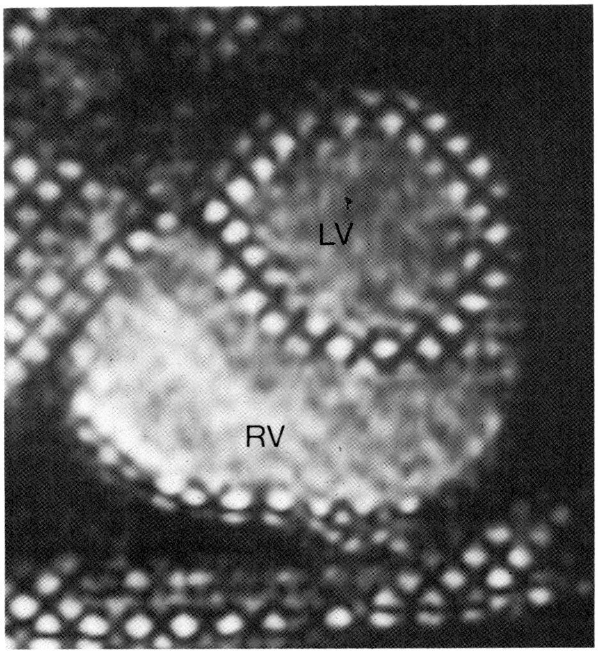

253, 254 Normal magnetic resonance image of the left ventricle (LV) in long axis (**253**) and short axis (**254**) views. These show the myocardium to be approximately 1.2 cm in thickness, which can be measured directly by the 8 mm grid on this image. This should be compared with **255** and **256**.

255, 256 Magnetic resonance scans in left ventricular hypertrophy using the same projections as the normal examples in **253** and **254**. One can see there is gross thickening of the ventricular walls and, since the grid remains 8 mm, the wall thickness exceeds 2.4 cm.

255

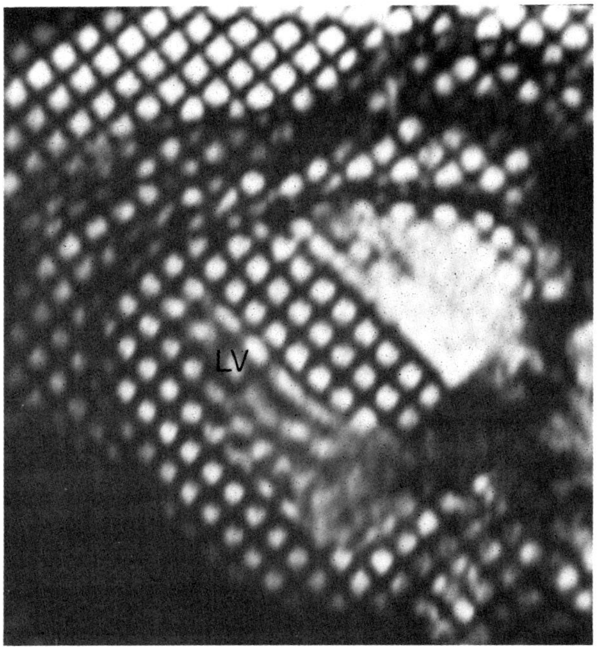

256

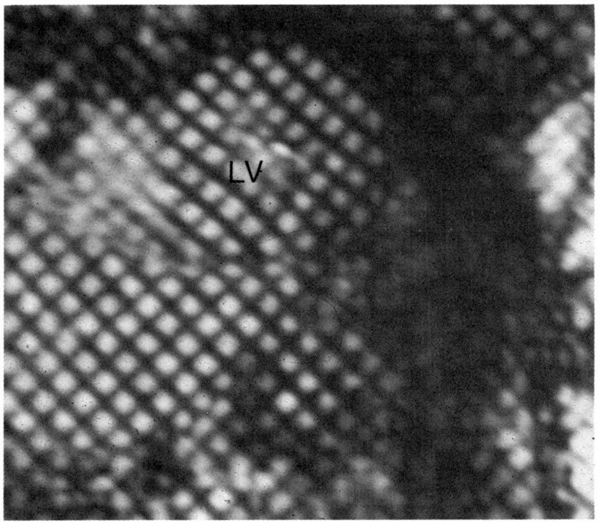

Congestive heart failure

The Framingham study demonstrated the clear relationship between hypertension and congestive heart failure. Of all the patients with congestive heart failure, 75% had predisposing hypertension, and the incidence of heart failure rose as systolic or diastolic pressure increased, irrespective of age or sex.

Hypertensive heart failure occurs almost invariably on the basis of poor systolic function of the left ventricle. Left ventricular systolic and diastolic volume increases, and poor function results in increasing left ventricular end diastolic pressure. Patients may be symptomatic in mild cases, with exertional breathlessness due to pulmonary congestion and poor cardiac output. As the heart failure worsens, dyspnoea at rest, fatigue and peripheral oedema may become the predominant features. The physical signs of heart failure include third and fourth heart sounds, small volume pulse, tachypnoea, tachycardia, raised venous pressure and peripheral oedema. Functional systolic murmurs of mitral regurgitation are not uncommon.

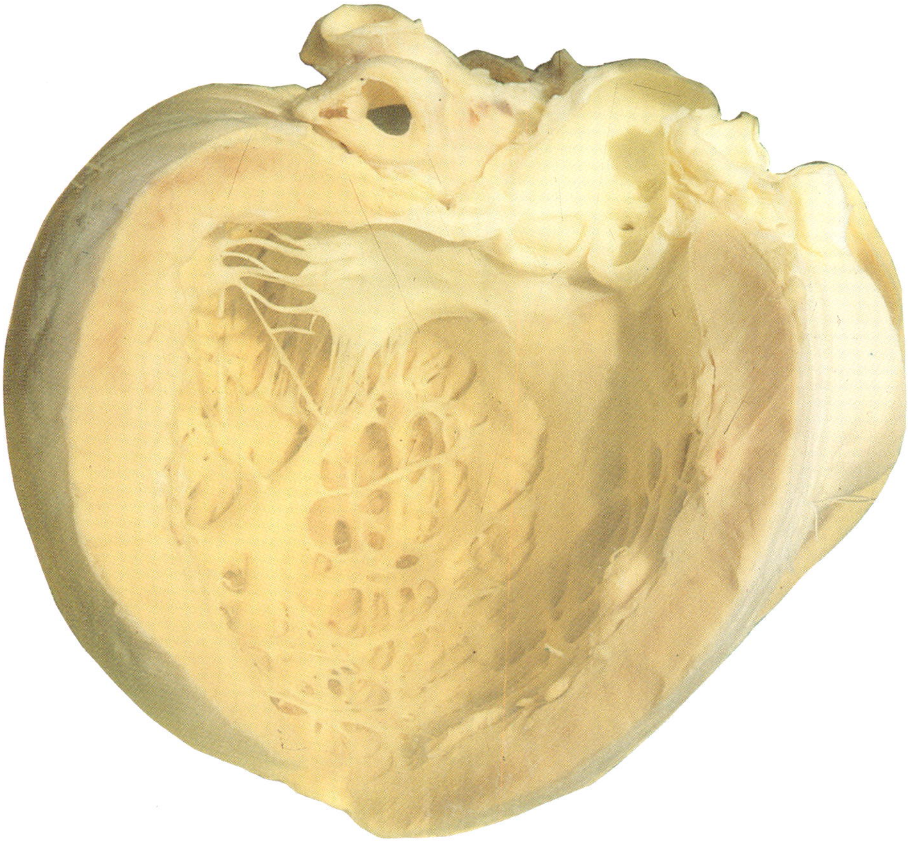

257

257 Pathological specimen in hypertensive heart failure showing a dilated, hypertrophied left ventricle.

258

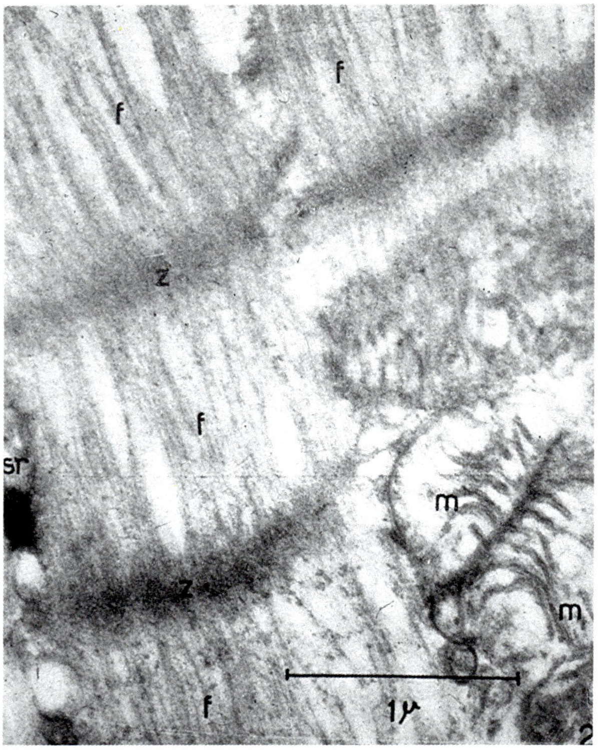

258 Electron microscopy of the myocardium in heart failure. The mitochondria are shown to be swollen and there are also degenerative changes. SR = sarcoplasmic reticulum; F = myofibril; Z = z bands; M = mitochondria.

259

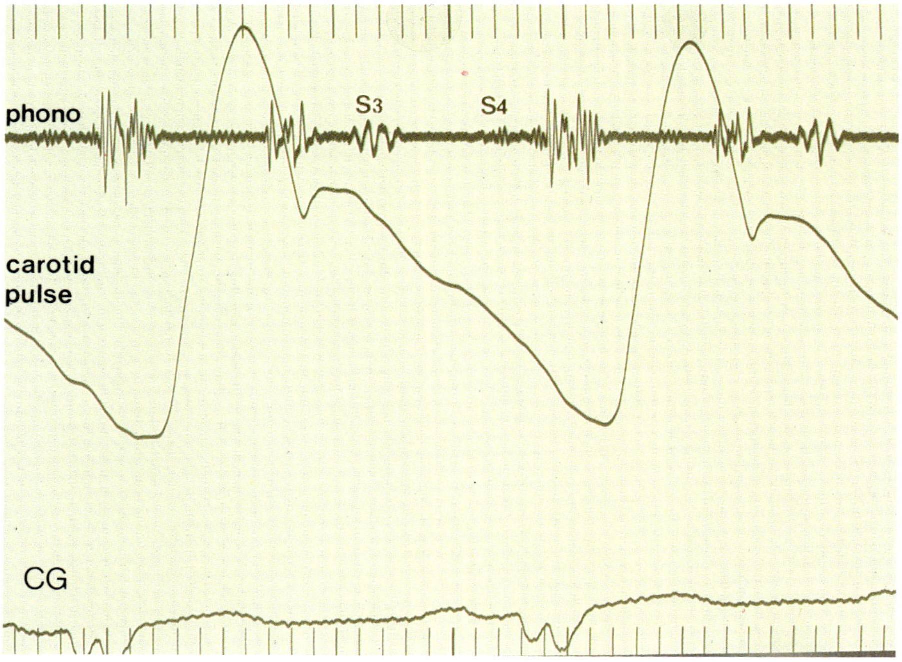

259 Physical signs in hypertensive heart failure showing third and fourth heart sounds, and an ill-sustained carotid pulse.

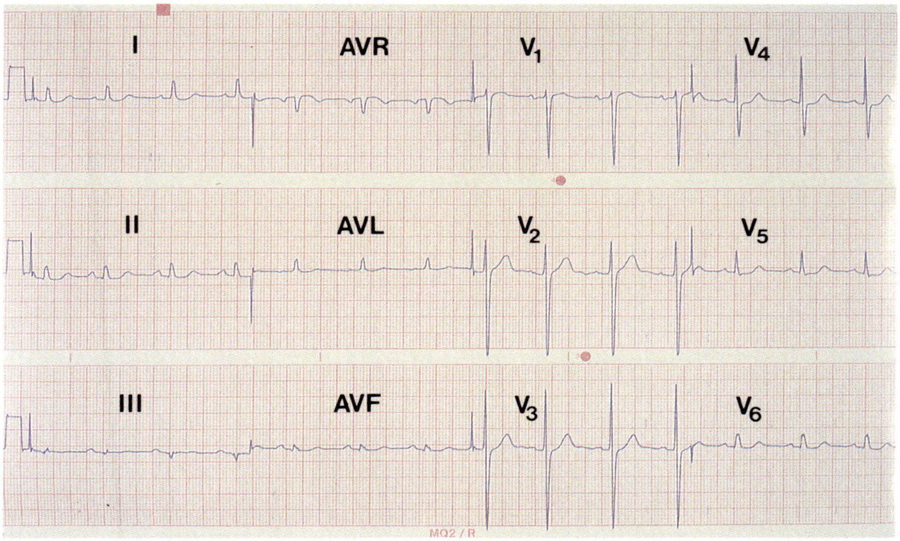

260

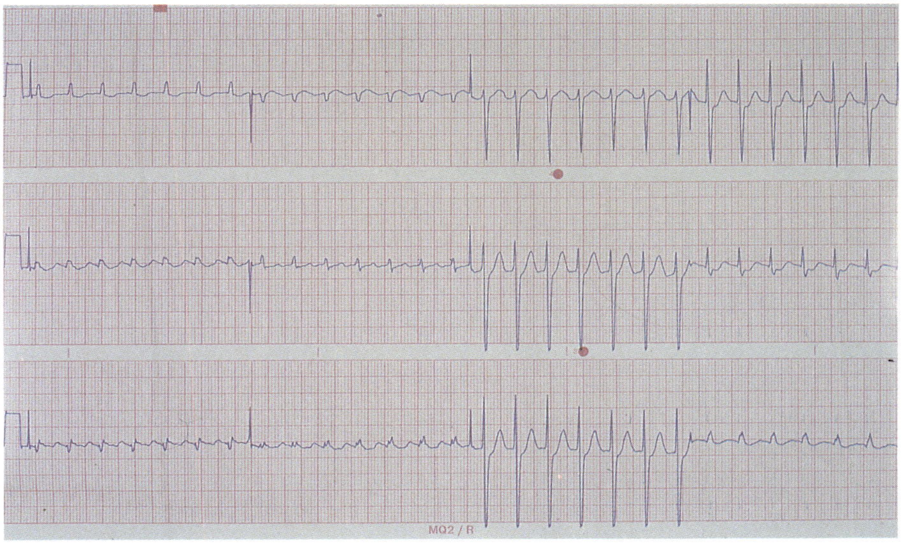

261

260, 261 Electrocardiogram in heart failure. Many patients with hypertension deteriorate markedly with the onset of atrial tachyarrhythmias. In **260**, the patient has left ventricular hypertrophy in sinus rhythm, but develops atrial flutter (**261**) with the onset of heart failure.

262

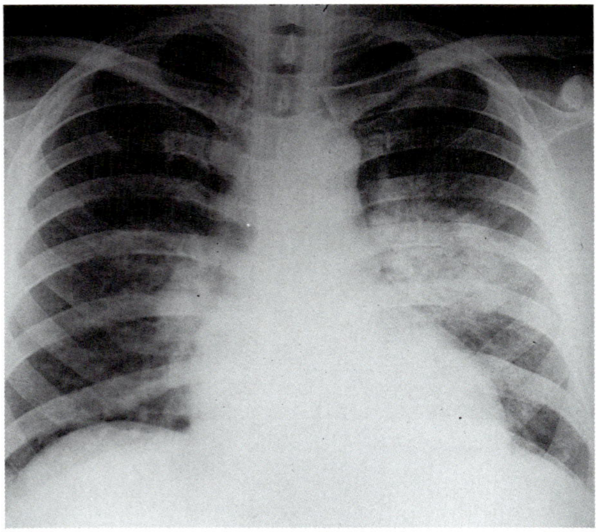

262 Chest radiograph in hypertensive heart disease showing a normal sized heart with pulmonary oedema.

263

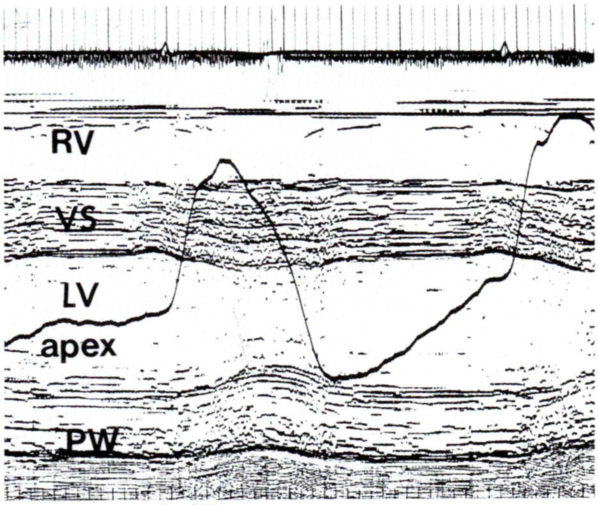

263, 264 Echocardiograms in hypertensive heart failure. The M-mode echocardiogram (**263**) shows grossly thickened myocardium with poor systolic contraction of the left ventricle (LV). The cross-sectional echocardiogram in the same patient (**264**), confirms the presence of symmetrical left ventricular hypertrophy.

264

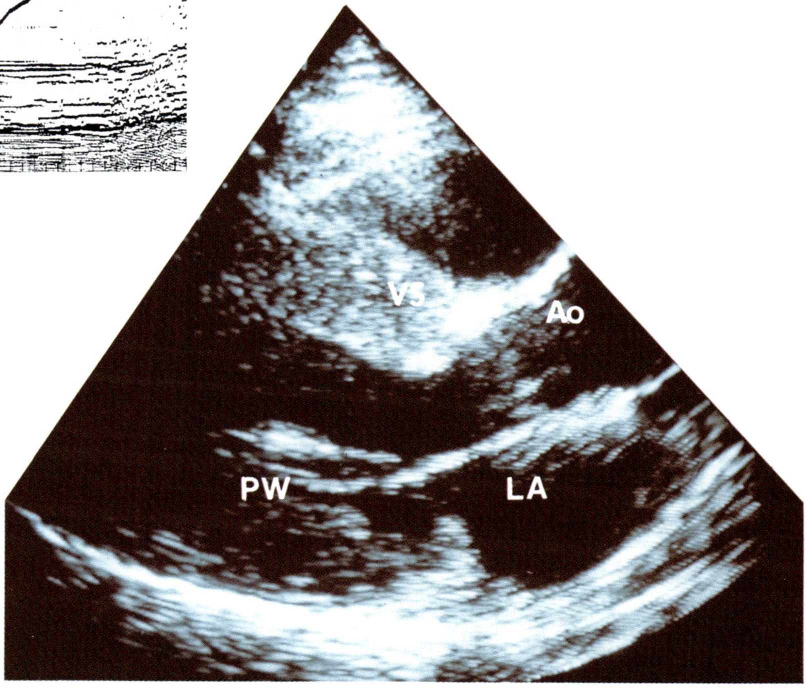

265

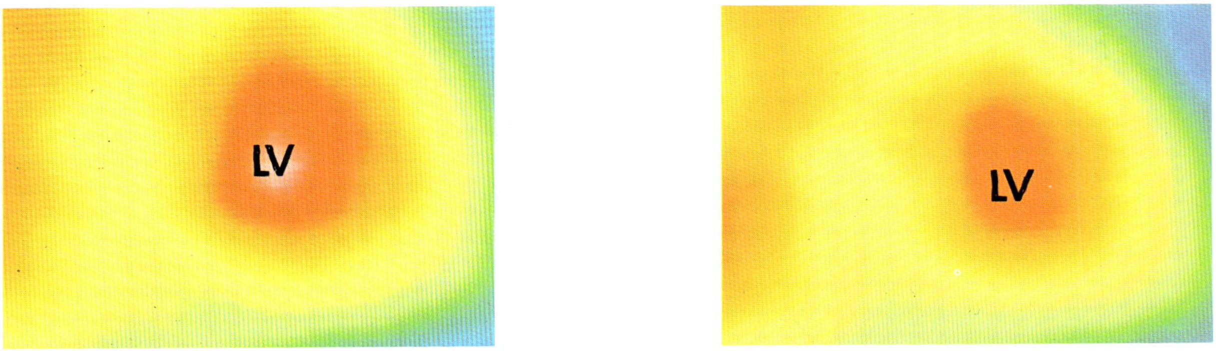

265 Gated blood pool scanning in diastole (left) and systole (right) in a patient with hypertensive heart failure. Only a small amount of contraction of the left ventricle is seen.

266

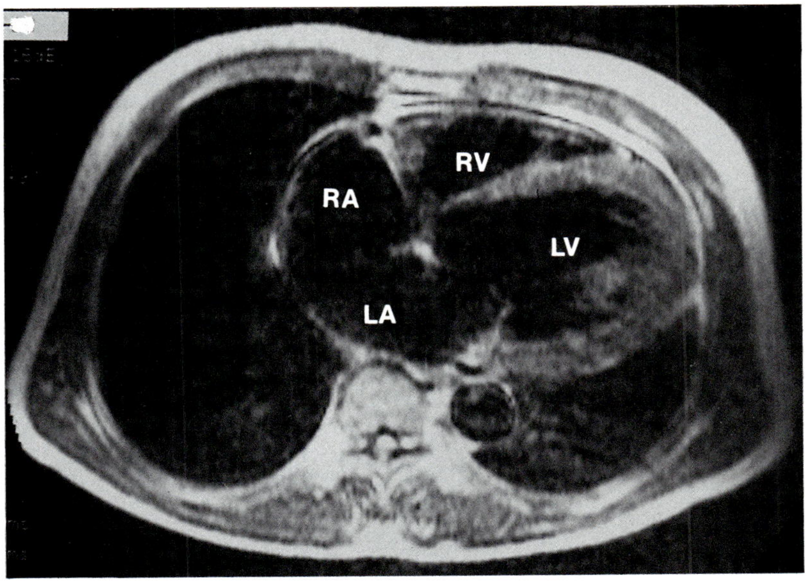

266 Magnetic resonance scan in transverse section through the heart in a patient with hypertensive heart failure. This shows a dilated left ventricle with moderate thickening of the ventricular wall. The degree of hypertrophy often appears less prominent than one may expect because thinning of the myocardium occurs as ventricular dilatation progresses.

267

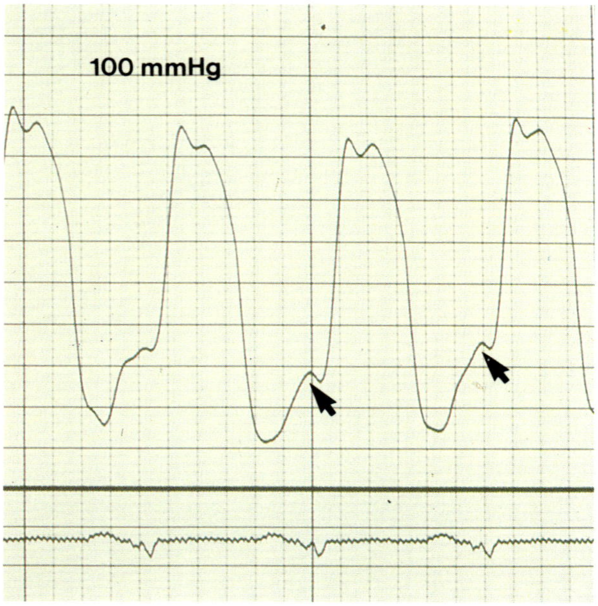

26

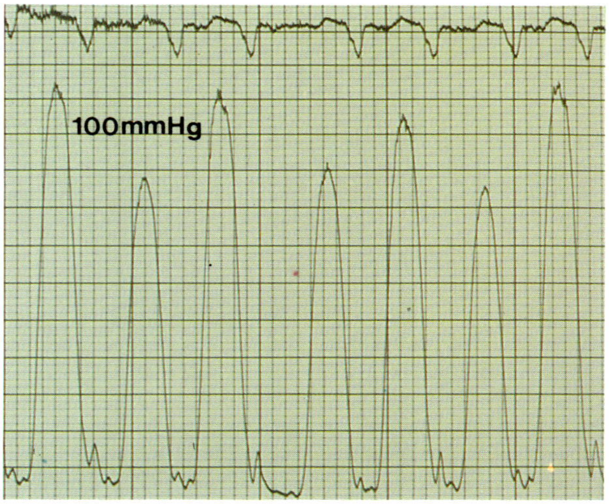

267 Left ventricular pressure trace showing an elevation of the left ventricular end diastolic pressure (arrow) in heart failure.

268 Pulsus alternans in a left ventricular pressure trace in a patient with hypertensive heart failure. Pulsus alternans is an ill-understood phenomenon that reflects severe impairment of left ventricular function in pressure-overloaded chambers.

269

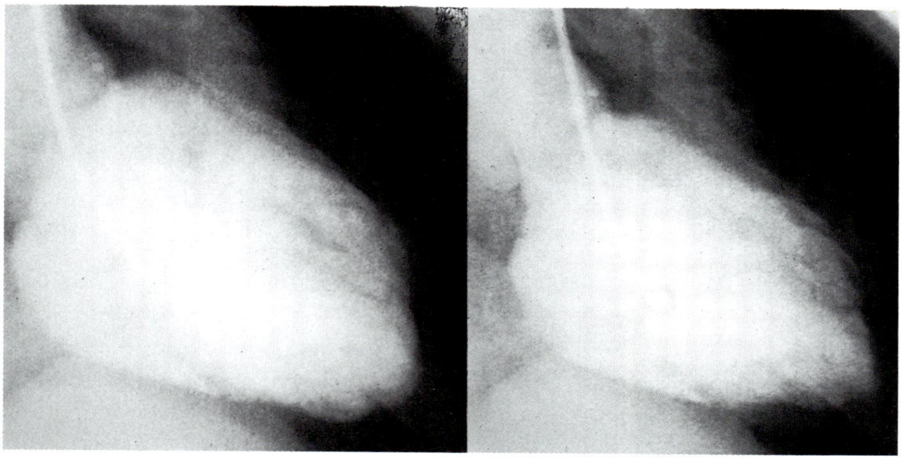

269 Left ventriculogram in systole (right) and diastole (left) showing a dilated, poorly functioning left ventricle.

Coronary artery disease

Hypertension may result in rapidly progressive coronary disease presenting as angina, myocardial infarction, or sudden death. The Framingham study showed that the incidence of myocardial infarction was almost twice as high among hypertensives as among normotensives. In addition, hypertensive patients have an increased risk of silent myocardial infarction. It may be noted that a proportion of hypertensive patients, following an infarction, become normotensive.

Coronary artery disease may be investigated using electrocardiography (both at rest and on exercise), radio-isotope techniques, magnetic resonance scanning, and angiography. The coronary artery disease seen in hypertensive patients is similar to that of normotensive patients. The management is also similar, except that in severely hypertensive patients, thrombolysis may need to be omitted during acute myocardial infarction.

270 Transverse ventricular section in an acute anteroseptal myocardial infarction. The infarcted area is haemorrhagic because the subtending coronary artery has been reperfused with streptokinase.

270

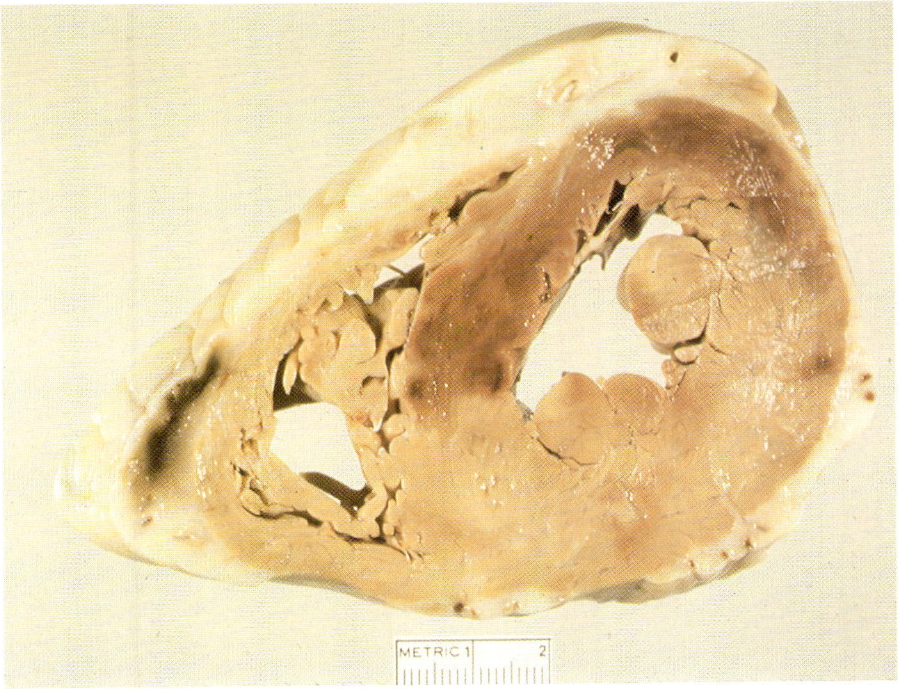

271

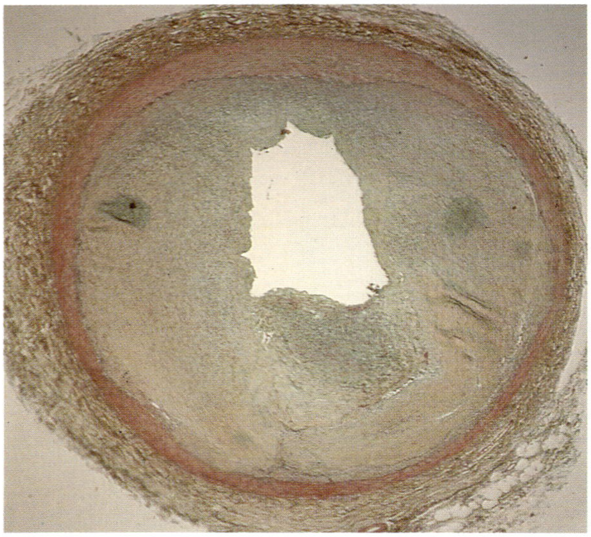

271, 272 Cross-sections of coronary arteries in atherosclerotic disease. **271** demonstrates a coronary artery that is narrowed by more than 75% in cross-sectional area by plaque. This significant degree of stenosis may lead to a reduction of myocardial blood flow and ischaemia. Disruption of the superficial layers of an atherosclerotic plaque by fissuring and intimal rupture leads to the passage of red blood cells into the plaque. Thrombus forms at this site and may become occlusive, as in this example (**272**).

272

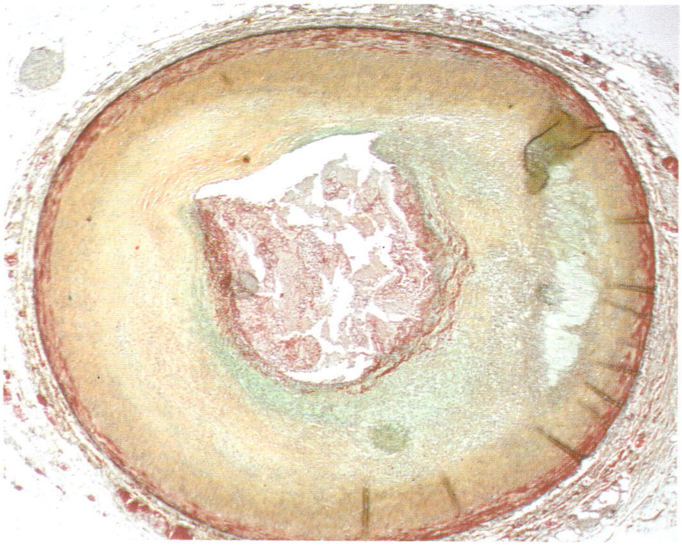

273

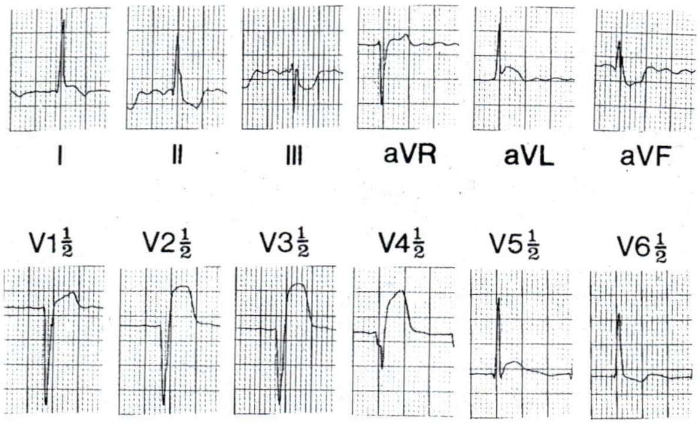

273 Twelve-lead electrocardiogram showing an acute anteroseptal myocardial infarction. This is demonstrated by Q-waves from V1 to V4 with ST segment elevation.

274–276 Exercise electrocardiography may be used to demonstrate the presence of myocardial ischaemia in hypertensive patients with coronary artery disease. **274** shows an essentially normal resting electrocardiogram with only minor inferolateral ST segment sagging. At Stage 3 of the Bruce protocol, a heart rate of 150 beats per minute is achieved, with marked lateral ST segment depression. This represents reversible myocardial ischaemia (**275**). **276** demonstrates computer-averaging of the resting and exercising electrocardiogram. The first beat in each pair from each of the leads represents the resting electrocardiogram, and the second that of the particular level of exercise. This trace was taken at the end of Stage I of the Bruce protocol and shows gross anterolateral ST segment depression with T-wave inversion. Such levels of ischaemia at low work loads represent severe underlying coronary artery disease.

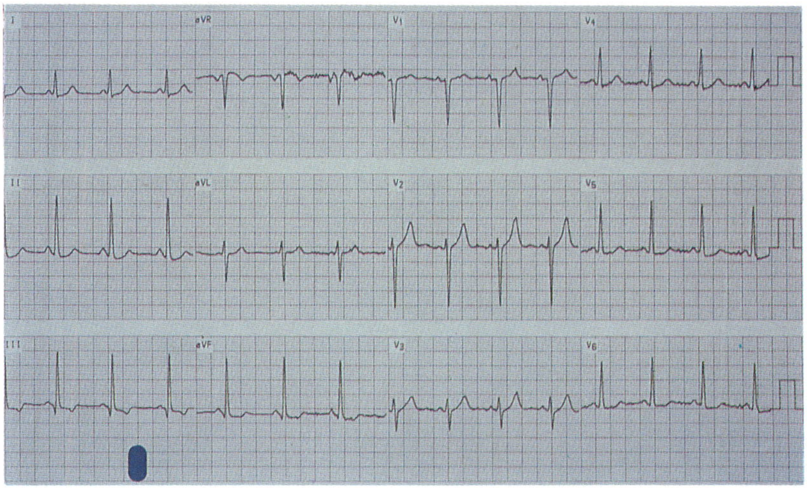

274

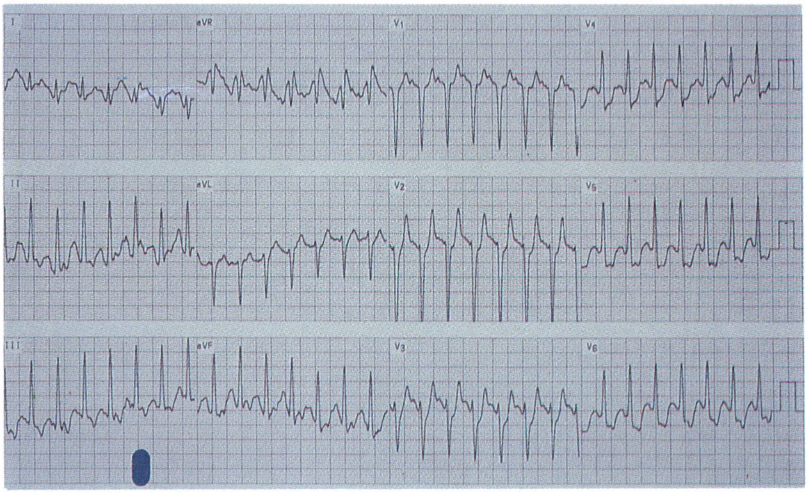

275

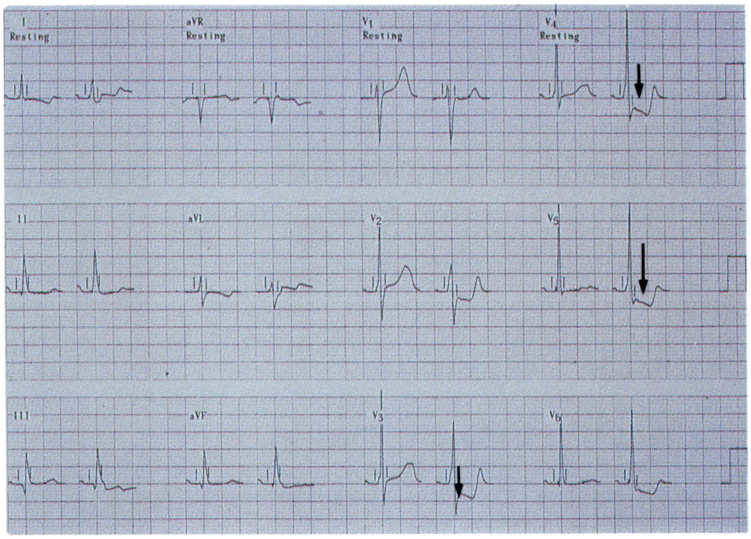

276

277

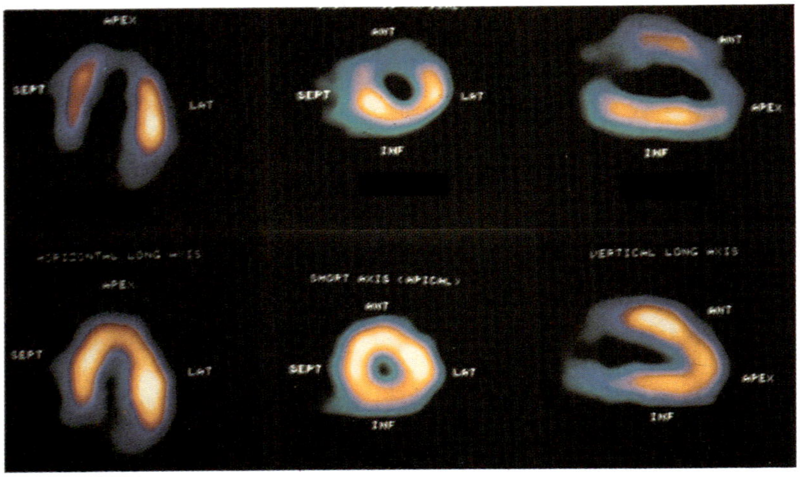

277 Thallium scintigraphy may be used at rest and exercise to demonstrate myocardial perfusion. This demonstrates a sequence of thallium tomograms with the stress images above and the rest images below, in three planes. There are defects in the septum, distal anterior wall, and apex. These defects returned to normal on the rest images.

278

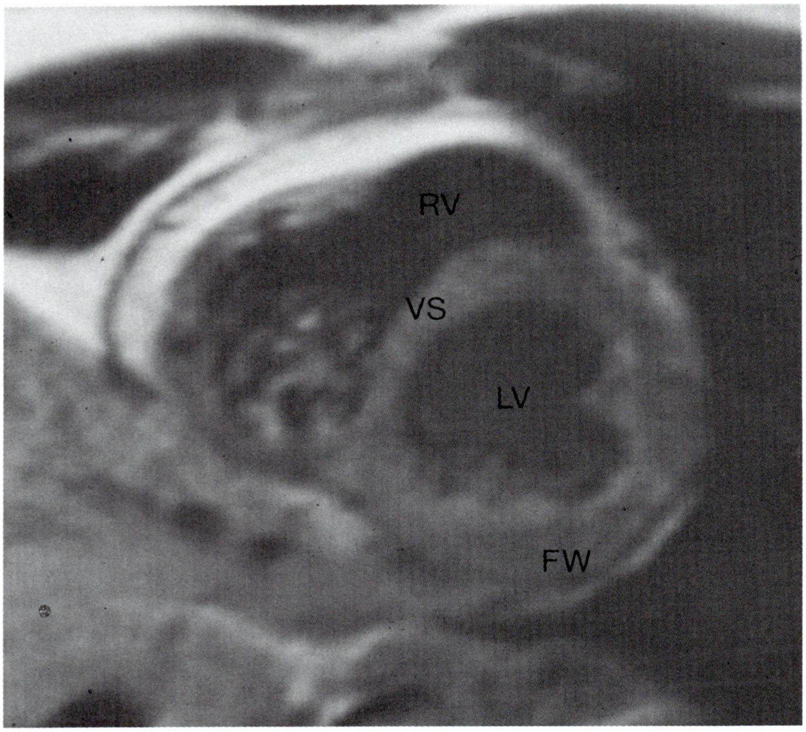

278 Magnetic resonance scan of the short axis of the left ventricle. This shows a hypertrophied free wall (FW) of the left ventricle with thinning of the septum (VS) and posterior lateral sections. Hypertrophy is both compensatory from the level of left ventricular damage, and due to hypertension. The area of thinning of the myocardium is clearly seen on this image.

279

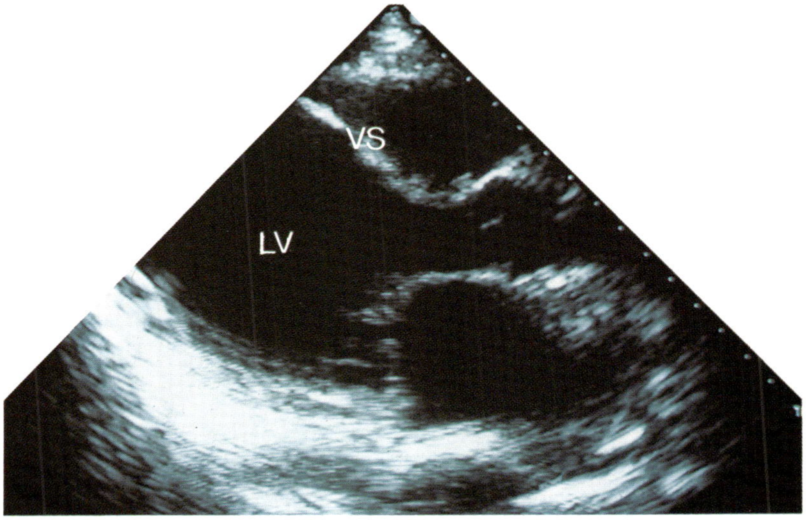

279 Cross sectional echocardiogram in a hypertensive patient following a septal myocardial infarction. The left ventricle (LV) is dilated and the septum (VS) thinned.

280

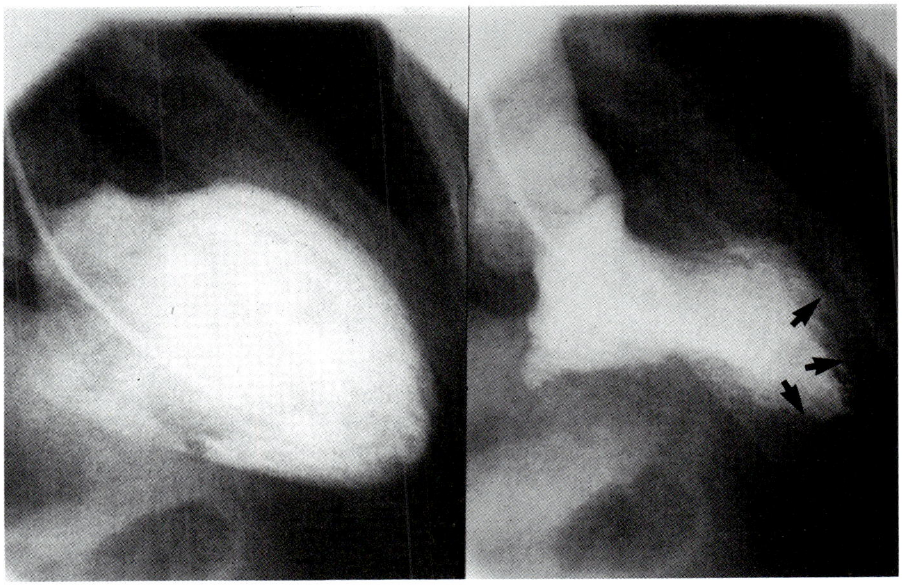

280 The contrast left ventriculogram, diastole (left) and systole (right), shows anterior and apical akinesis in a patient with an old anterior–apical infarction.

281

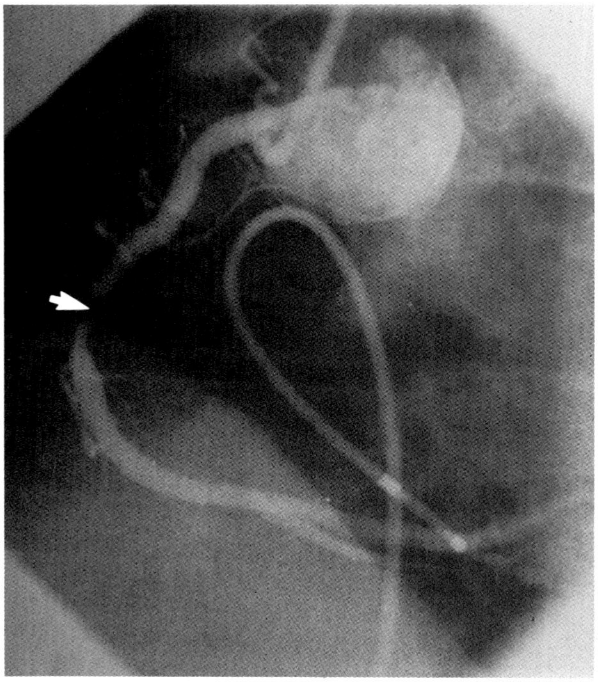

28

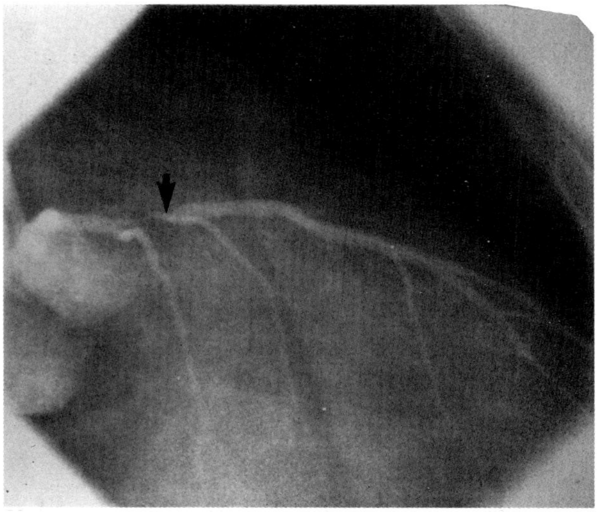

28

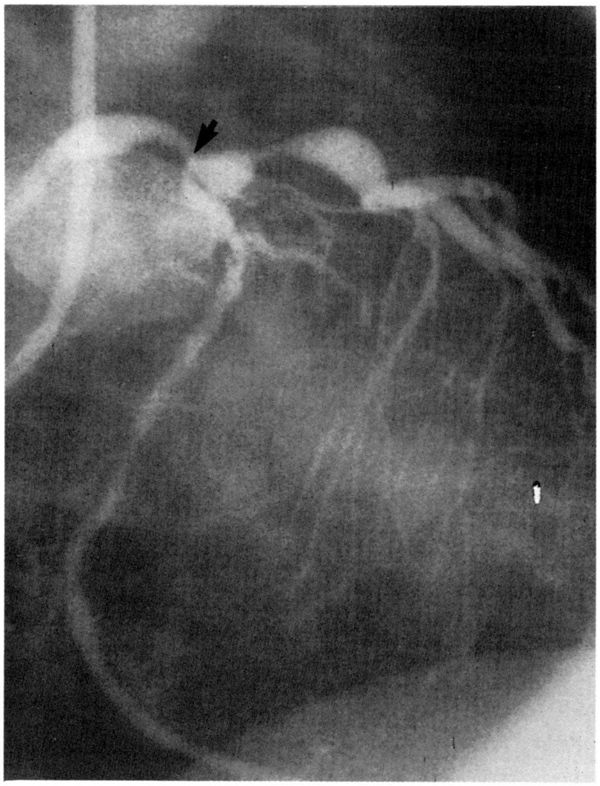

283

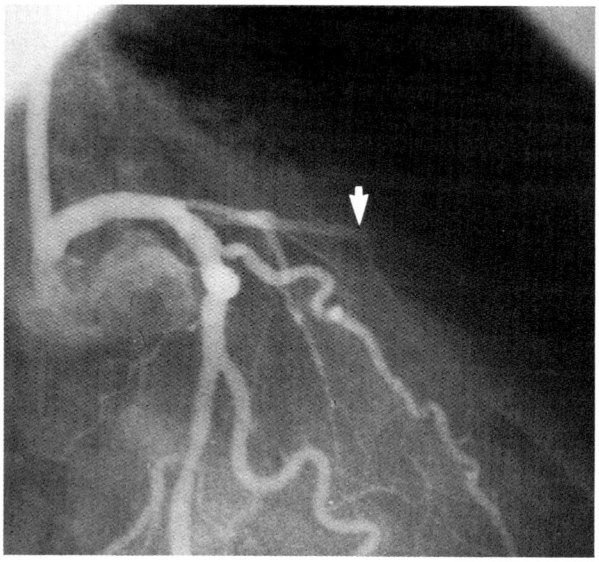

281–284 Coronary arteriography remains the method of choice for demonstrating coronary arterial anatomy. The right coronary artery shows a mid-vessel stenosis (**281**, arrow). The left anterior descending coronary artery is shown both stenosed (**282**) and occluded proximally (**283**). The left main stem coronary artery disease is the most significant prognostic lesion (**284**).

Vascular complications of hypertension

Peripheral vascular disease

Occlusive atherosclerotic vascular disease of peripheral arteries is more common in patients with hypertension. Accelerated atherosclerosis and medial necrosis are probably predisposing factors for aortic aneurysm formation and aortic dissection. In the aorta, the lesions of atherosclerosis have a characteristic distribution. There may be a few plaques around the arch, but the lesions usually increase in concentration and severity along the course of the aorta towards the bifurcation. In the most severe cases, they may be confluent below the level of the renal arteries and, in this region, ulceration, mural thrombosis, and aneurysms may present as complications. Plaques may also form around the orifices of the side branches.

Patients may present with the symptoms of their peripheral vascular disease, for example, intermittent claudication, but in many others, it will be just a feature noted on examination with reduced peripheral pulses. In addition, the treatment of hypertension with beta-blockade may unmask the symptoms of intermittent claudication.

285

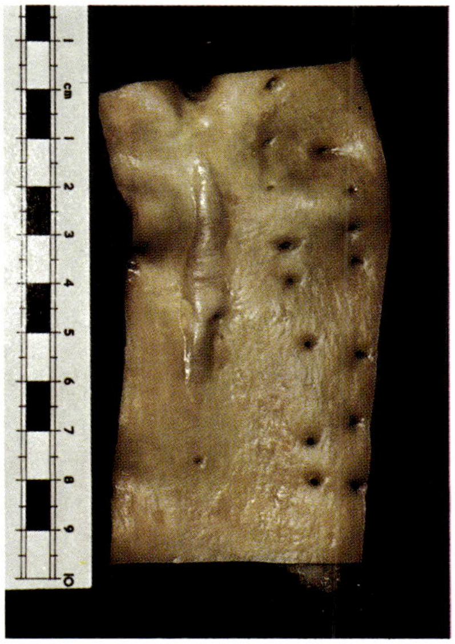

285 Pathology of atheroma. This portion of aorta from a young man is opened in the area of the intercostal arteries and shows an elevated fibrous plaque in the thoracic aorta.

286 Pathology of atheroma. Ulcerated complicated lesion of advanced atherosclerosis in the aorta with thrombus.

286

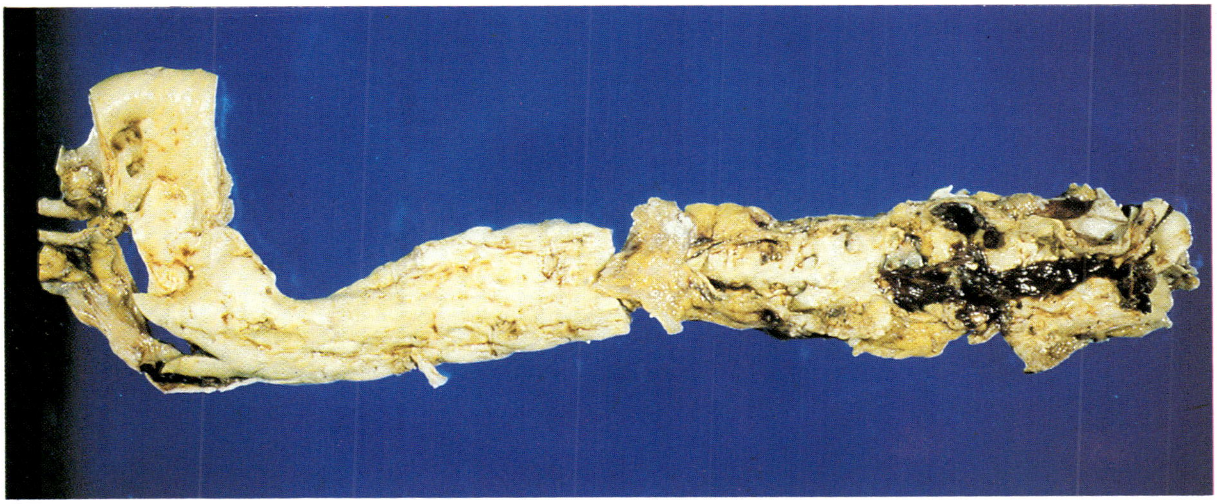

287

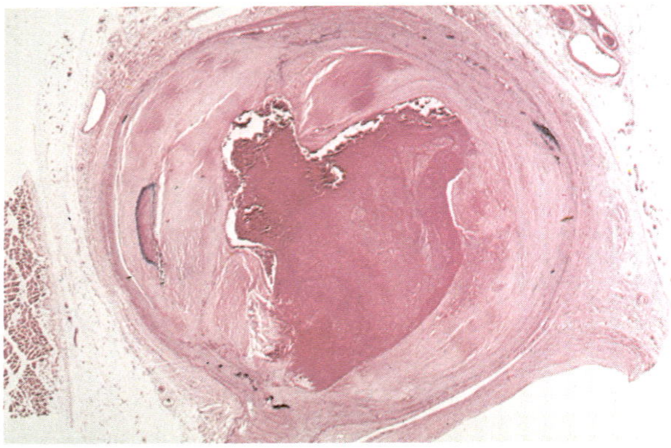

287 Histology of atheroma with recent thrombotic occlusion. There is circumferential thickening of the intima, patchy calcification of the plaques and marked atrophy of the media of the femoral artery from a patient with gangrene of the left foot and leg. The lumen is filled with recent thrombus in which atheromatous debris is present (H & E × 3).

288

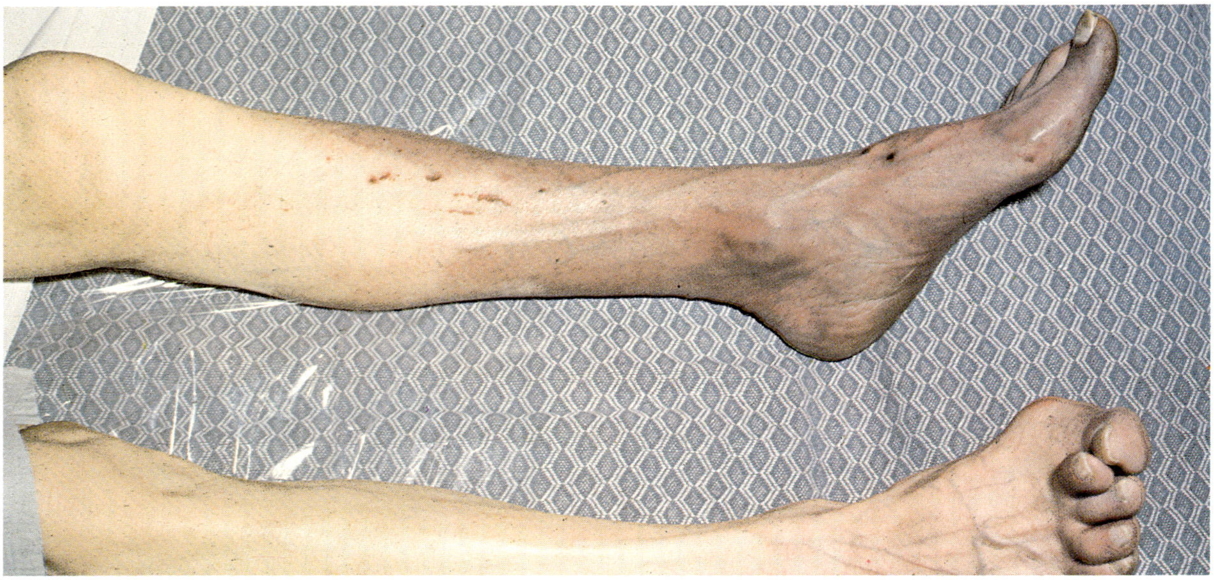

288 Clinical photograph of an ischaemic foot due to peripheral vascular disease. There is acute gangrene of the left leg due to thrombotic occlusion of an atherosclerotic popliteal artery.

289, 290 Doppler study of both lower limbs showing the normal (**289**) and markedly abnormal (**290**) waveforms, the latter being suggestive of bilateral iliac stenoses.

289

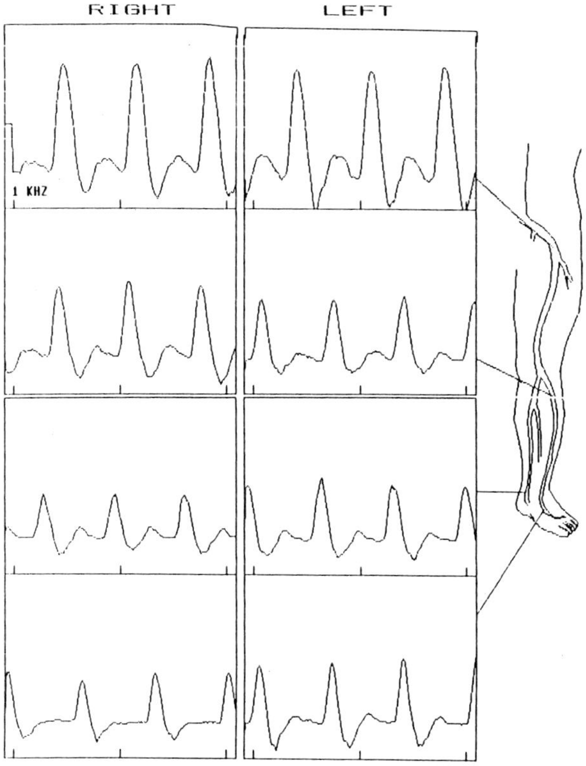

290

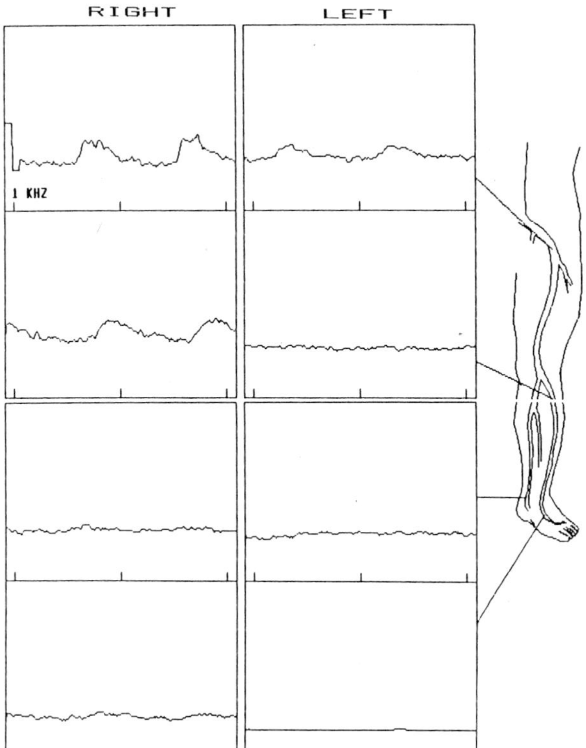

291

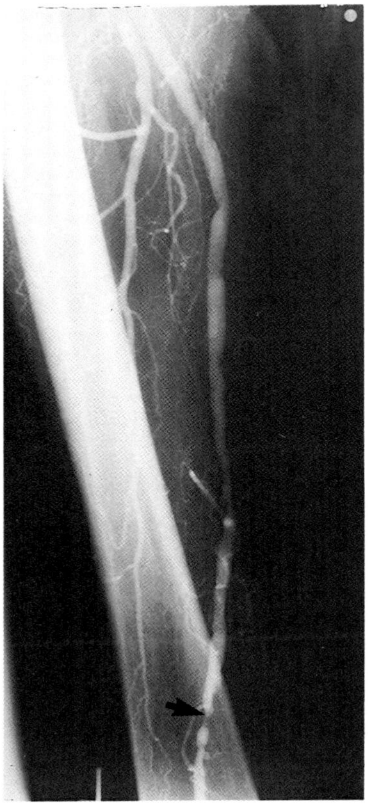

291–293 Angiography of affected arteries remains the method of choice for diagnosing both the extent and severity of peripheral vascular disease. This example shows extensive stenoses in the femoropopliteal system in the left leg (**291**). Complete occlusion of the popliteal artery (**292**) and bifurcation of the aorta (Ao, **293**) may also be demonstrated.

292

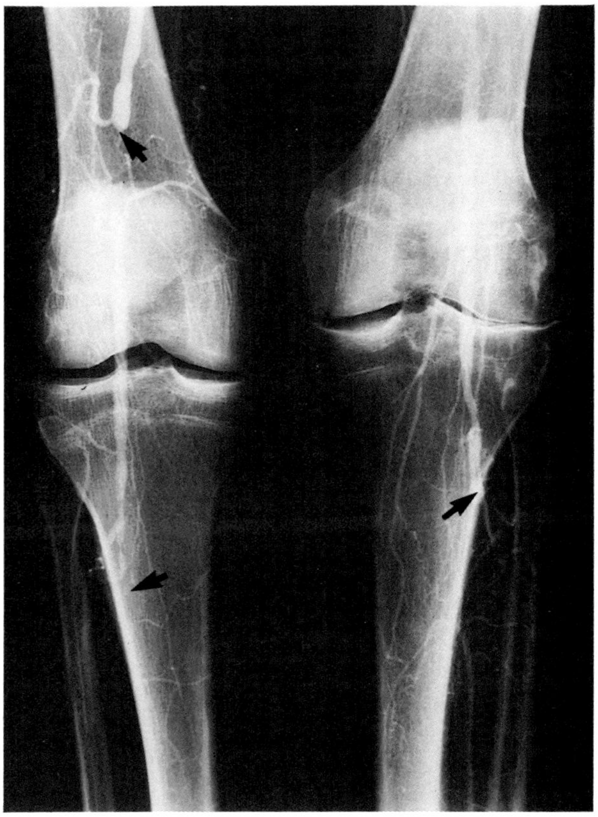

293

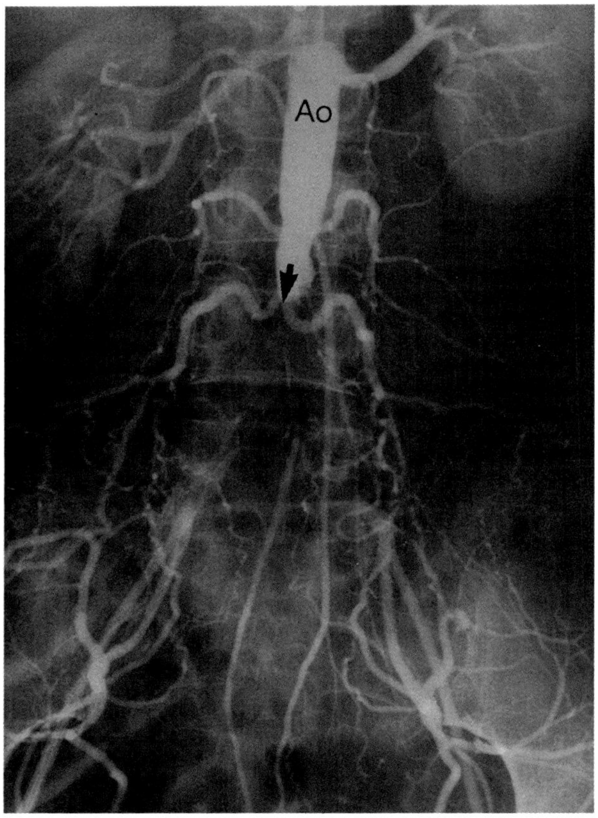

294 CT scans may show heavy calcification in an aorta (Ao) with diffuse atherosclerosis.

294

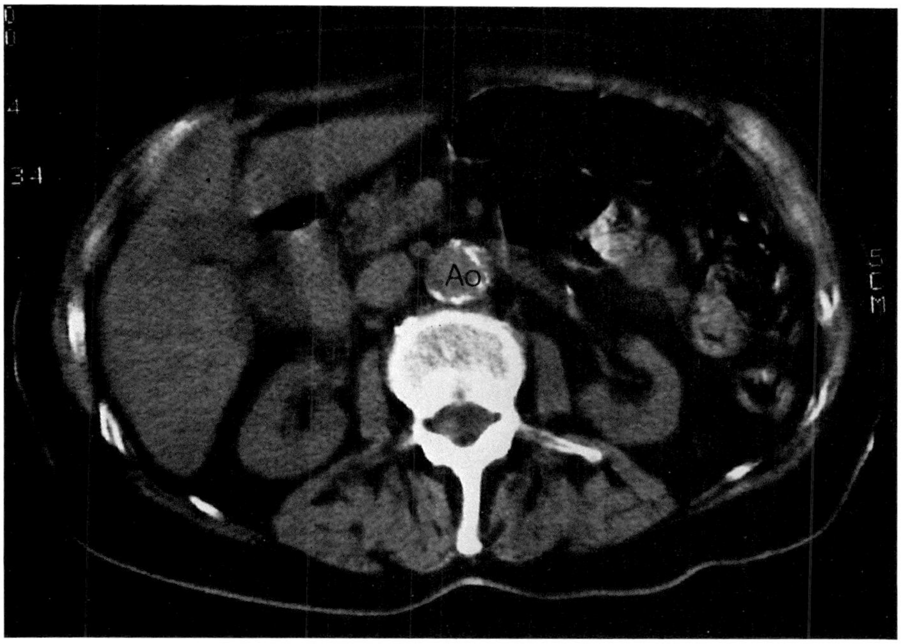

Aortic aneurysm

Acquired diseases of the aorta are primarily the result of degenerative changes in the aortic wall. Hypertension and atherosclerosis are prominent among the factors that lead to this degeneration. Experimentally, hypertension leads to structural aortic changes that accelerate medial degeneration. Hypertension may also decrease the blood flow in the vaso-vasorum, causing ischaemia of the aortic wall. Approximately three-quarters of aortic aneurysms are abdominal, with the remainder within the thoracic aorta.

295

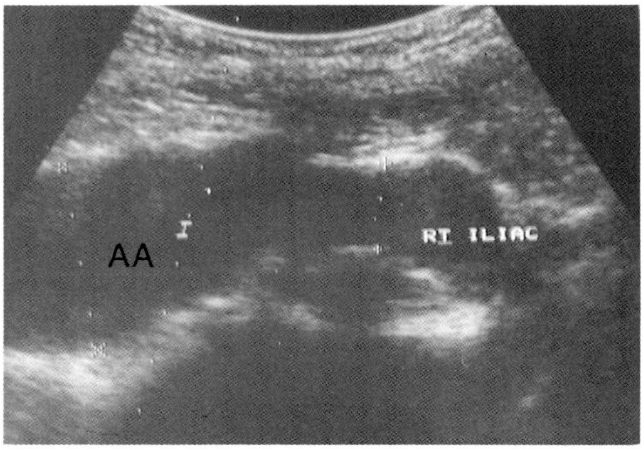

29

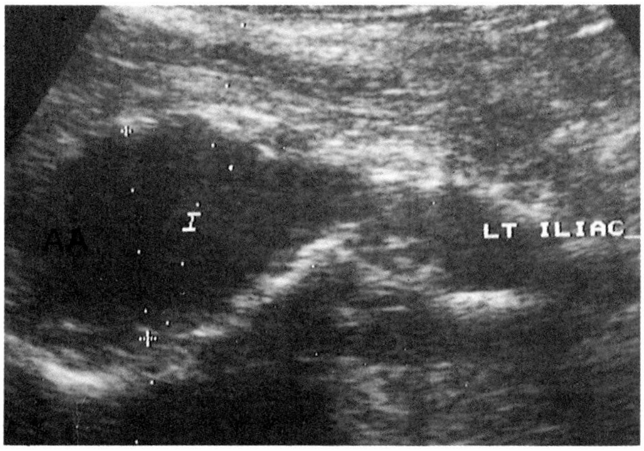

295, 296 Ultrasound scans of the descending aorta showing an aneurysmal dilatation (AA) above the bifurcation extending into the right (**295**), but not the left (**296**) iliac arteries.

97

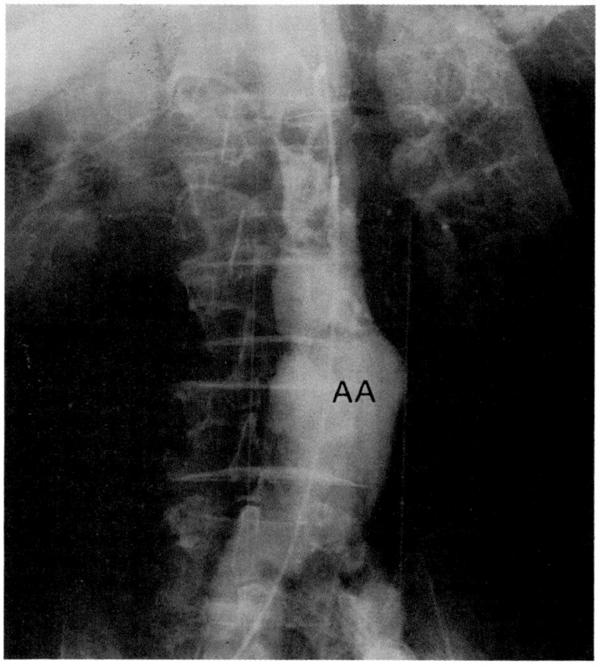

298

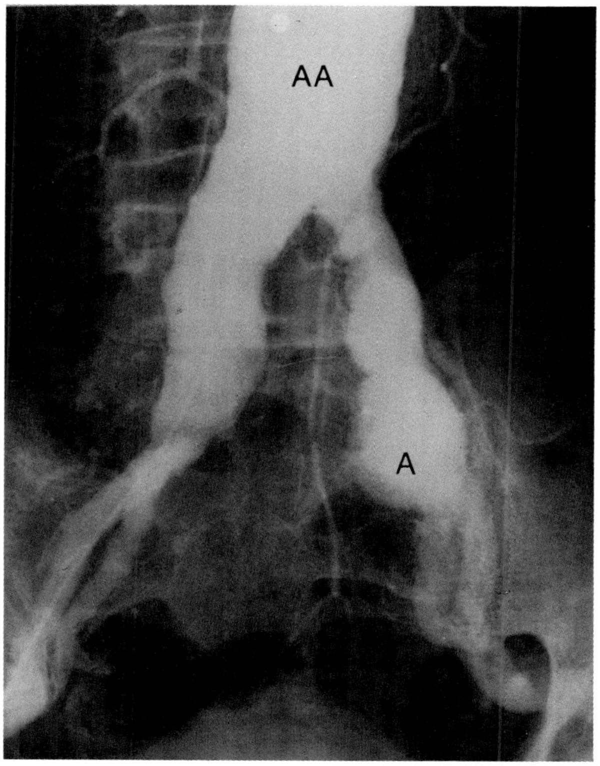

297, 298 Descending aortogram showing aneurysmal dilatation of both the aorta (AA) above the bifurcation (**297**) and the left common iliac artery (A, **298**).

99

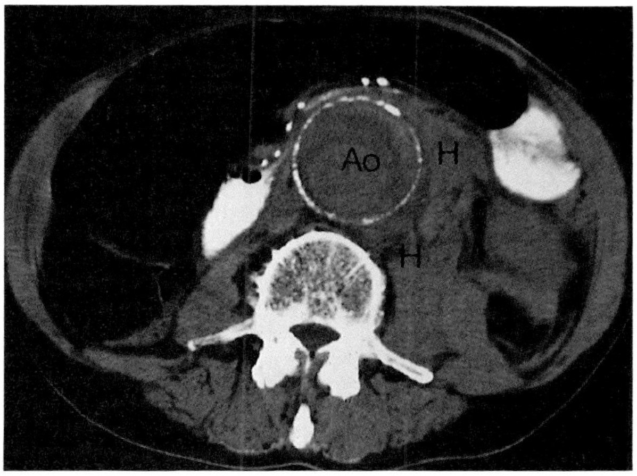

300

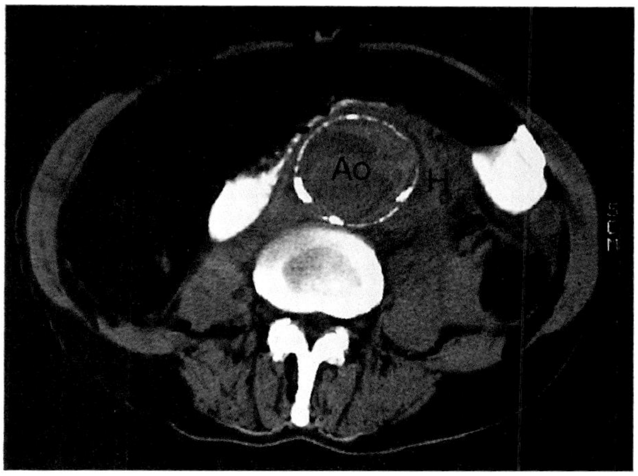

299, 300 CT scan of the same patient in **297** and **298** showing a dilated and calcified aorta (Ao) with haemorrhage (H) into the surrounding tissues.

301

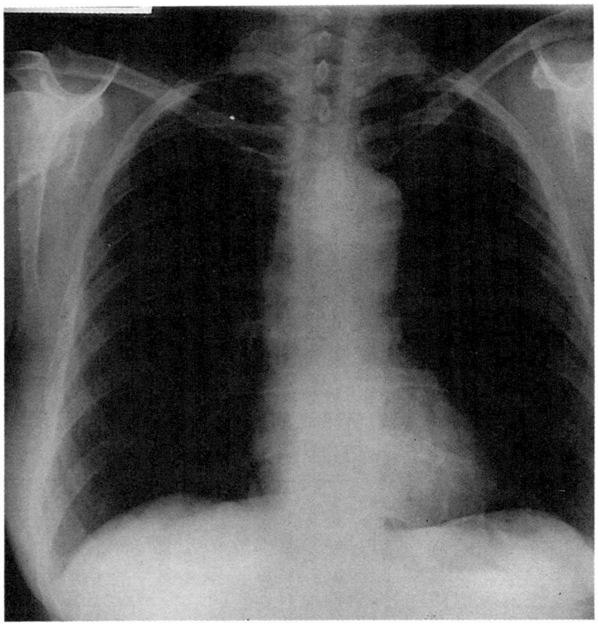

30

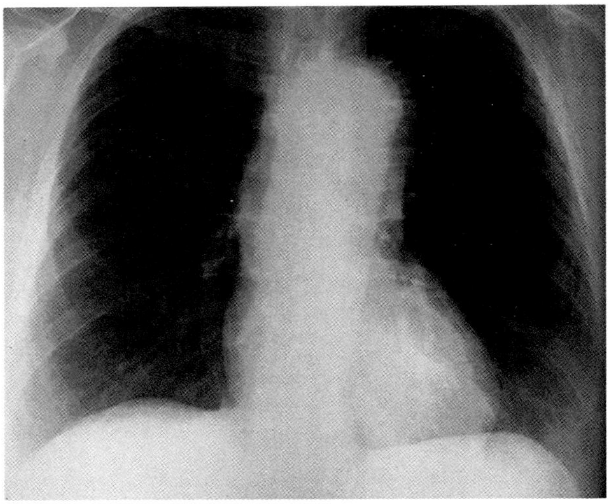

303

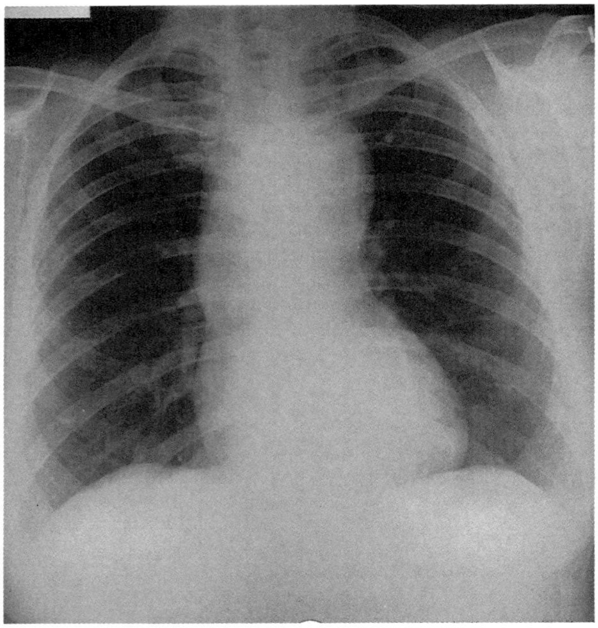

30

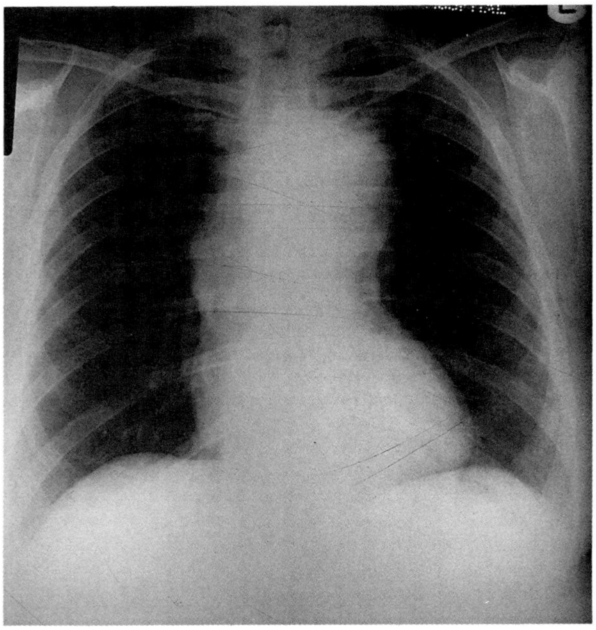

301–304 Development of a thoracic aortic aneurysm. A series of chest radiographs over a five-year period with progressive enlargement of the aortic silhouette. Compare these radiographs with the CT scans in **305–307**.

305–307 CT scans two years apart also demonstrate the progressive aortic enlargement (**305, 306**). Aortography shows gross aneurysmal dilatation in the arch of the aorta (**307**).

305

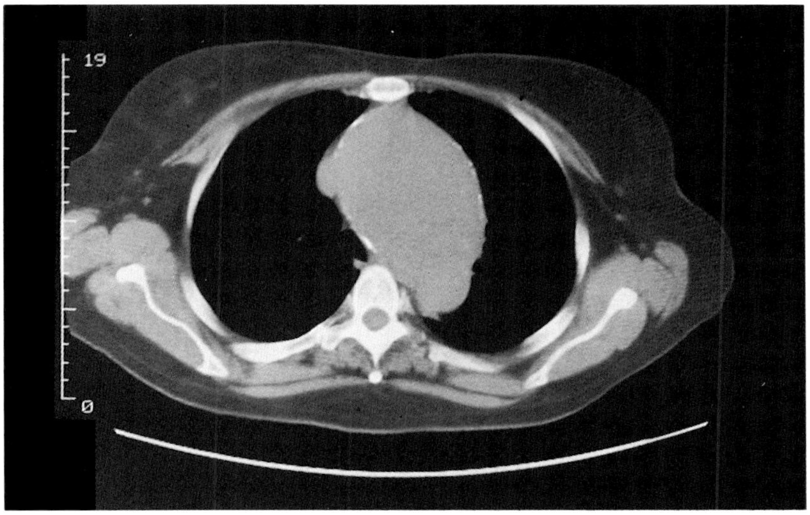

306

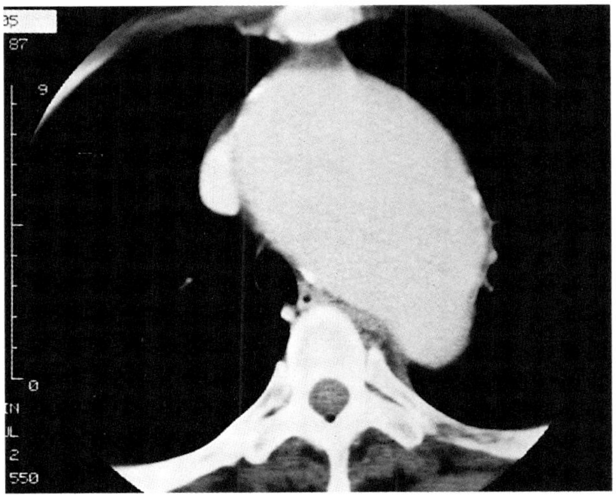

307

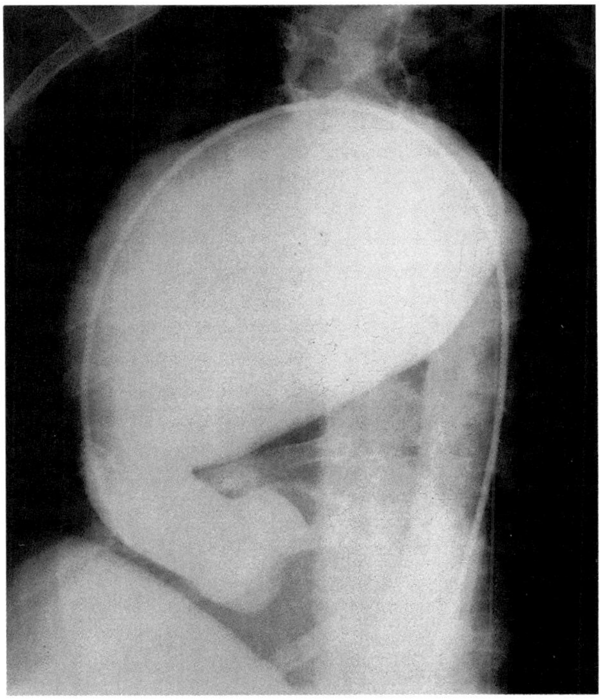

Aortic dissection

Aortic dissection is not an uncommon cause of acute catastrophic illness and sudden death. Acute aortic dissection is caused by the development of a tear in the aortic intima, allowing a column of blood driven by arterial pressure to enter the aortic wall, stripping the intima from the media.

Aortic medial degeneration is thought to be the underlying factor in the development of aortic dissection. Deterioration of the connective tissue, often with cystic changes, may be found. This is termed cystic medial necrosis and results from chronic aortic wall stress, particularly in hypertensive patients. However, this may also occur in connective tissue diseases, such as Marfan's syndrome. Well over half the patients with aortic dissection are hypertensive.

Aortic dissection is twice as common in men as in women, and most frequently affects individuals in their sixth and seventh decade. Severe pain, which is most marked at its onset, is the usual presenting feature. Painless dissection may rarely occur. Quality of the pain is often described as ripping or tearing and may move in its site of maximal intensity. Vasovagal symptoms are also common. The pain is often in the anterior chest radiating through to the back. Patients with dissection of the aorta may have no physical findings or present with shock or loss of arterial pulses. Development of aortic regurgitation or aortic tamponade may suggest the presence of ascending aortic dissection.

308

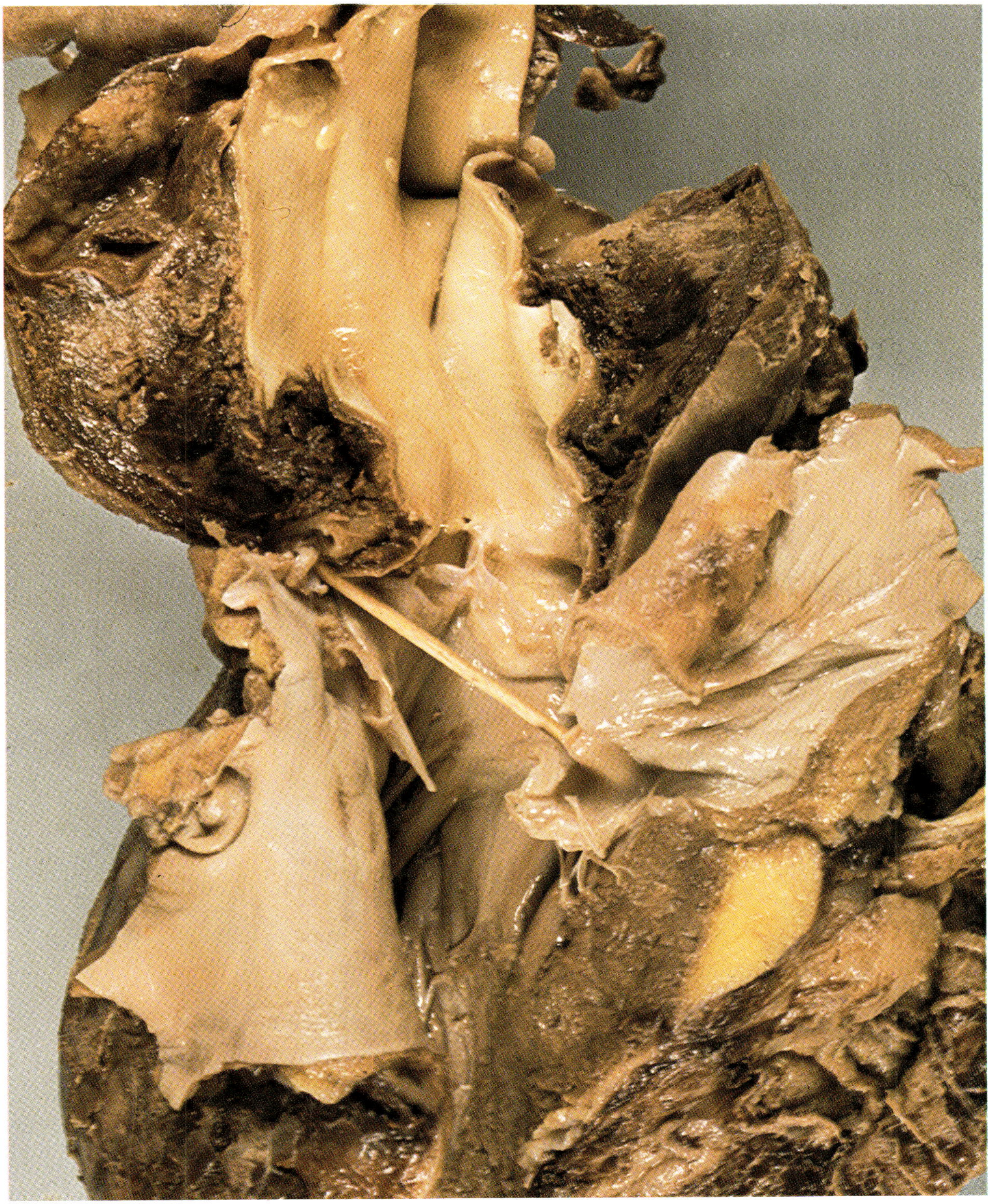

308 Shows a dilated aorta surrounded by a large haematoma in a false lumen. The intimal flap is marked.

309

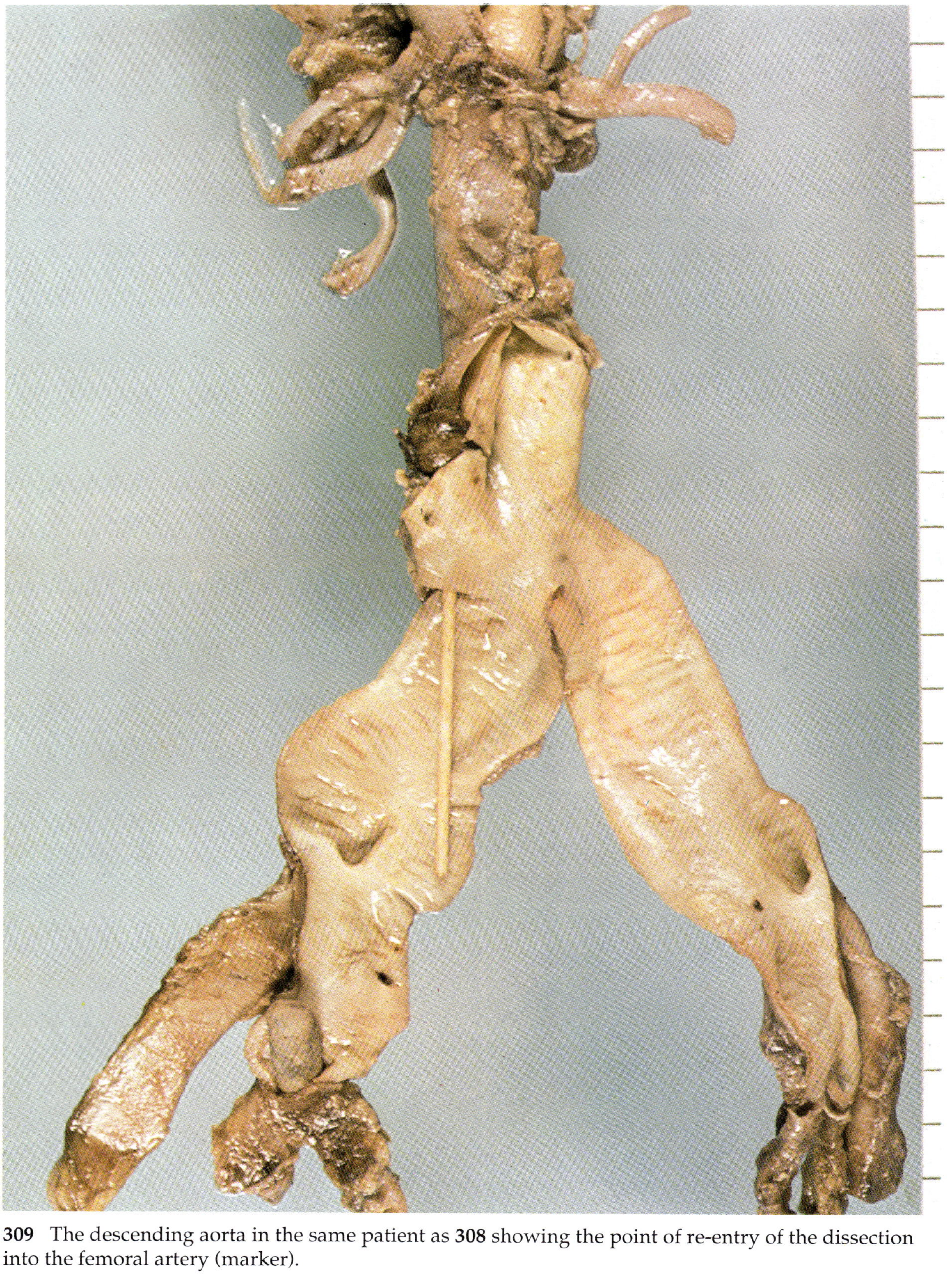

309 The descending aorta in the same patient as **308** showing the point of re-entry of the dissection into the femoral artery (marker).

310

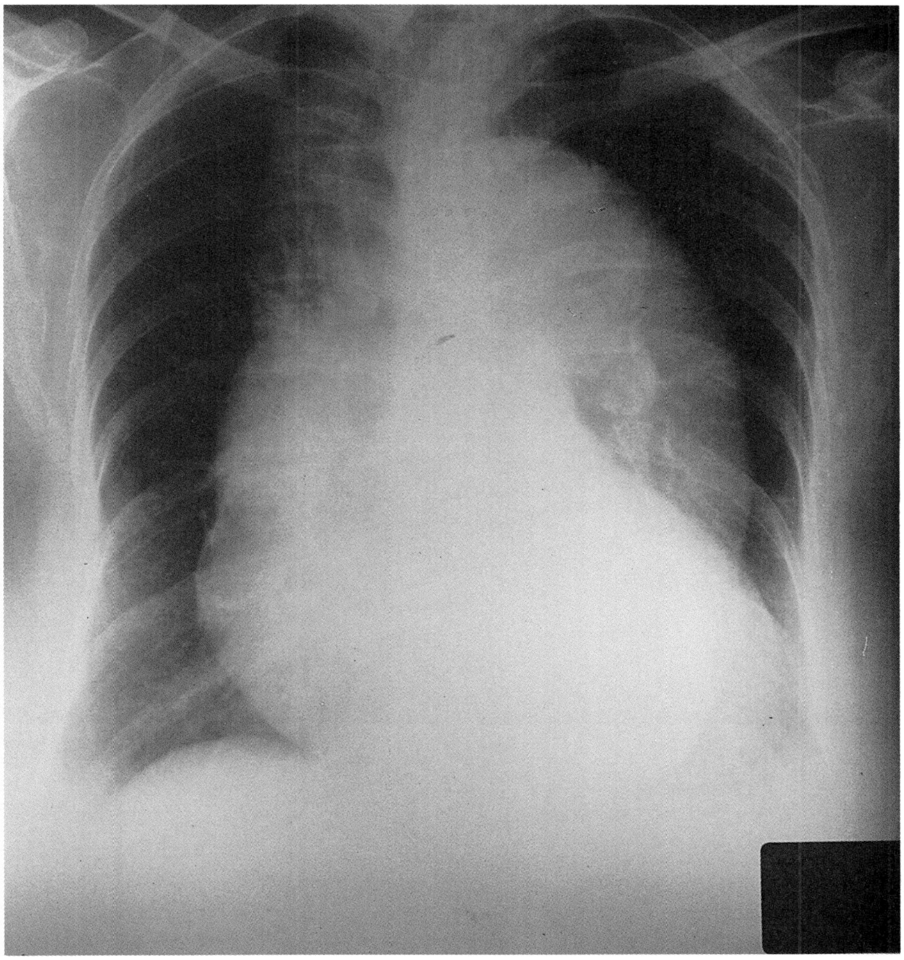

310 Chest radiograph in aortic dissection. This shows cardiomegaly and a huge aorta with a small left pleural effusion.

311

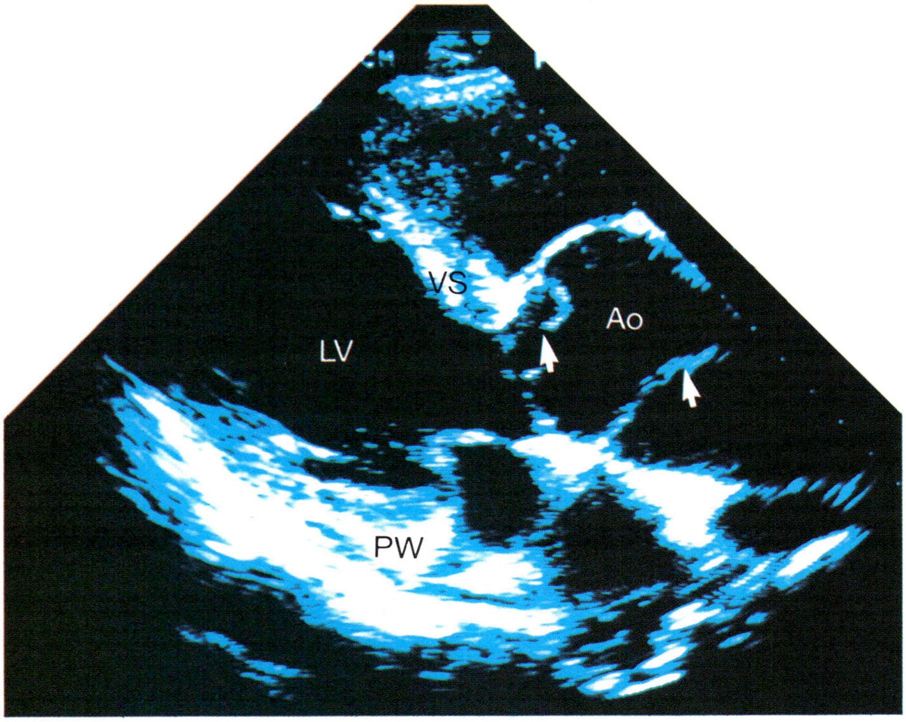

311 Echocardiogram in a dissection of the aorta. In this parasternal long axis view, the anterior and posterior intimal flaps of the dissection are clearly seen (arrows).

312

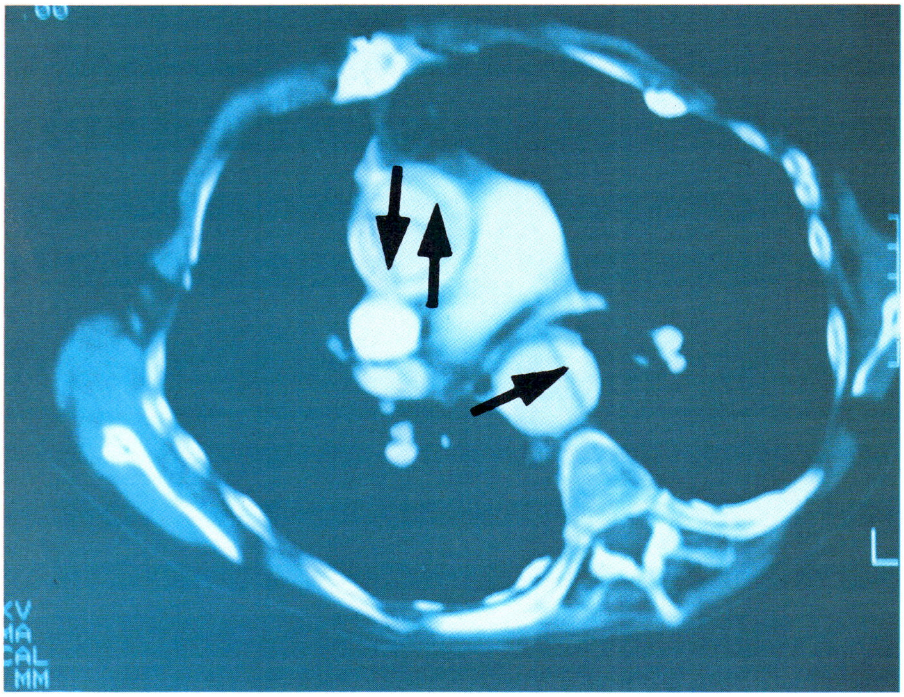

312 CT scan of an aortic dissection in a patient with hypertension. There are intimal flaps (arrowed) seen in the ascending and descending aorta.

313 Angiogram in a dissecting aortic aneurysm. An intimal flap is seen in the ascending aorta.

313

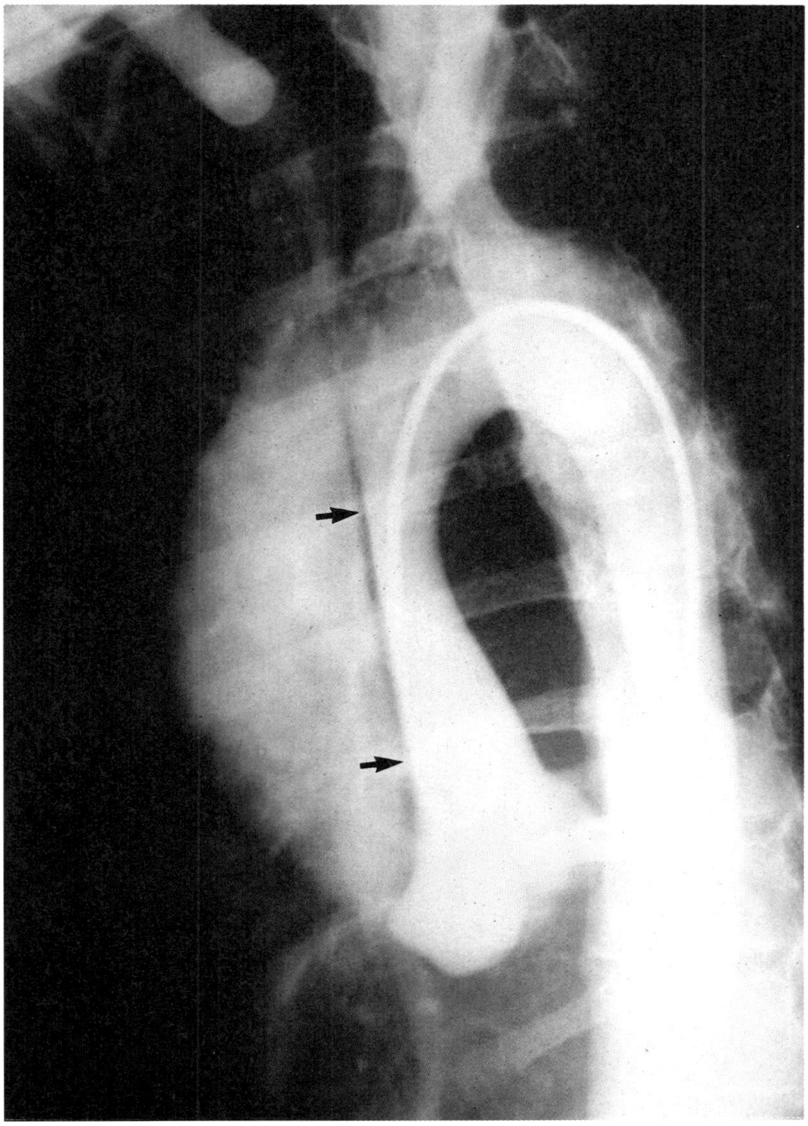

314 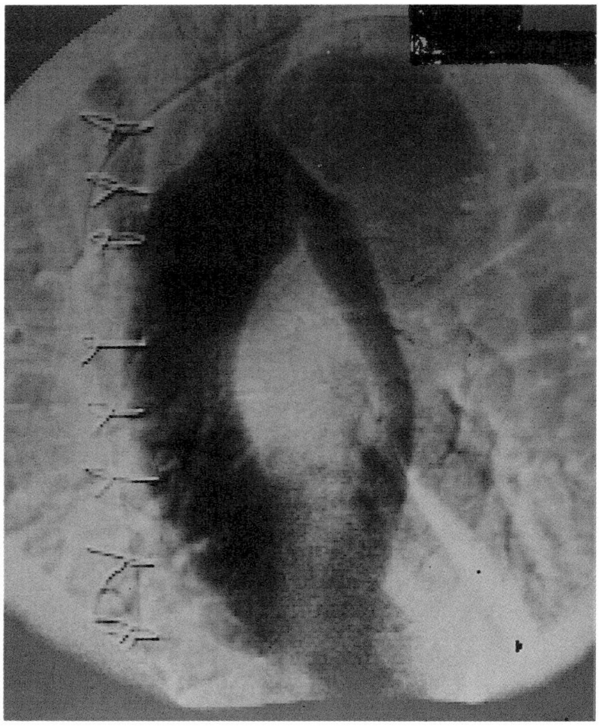

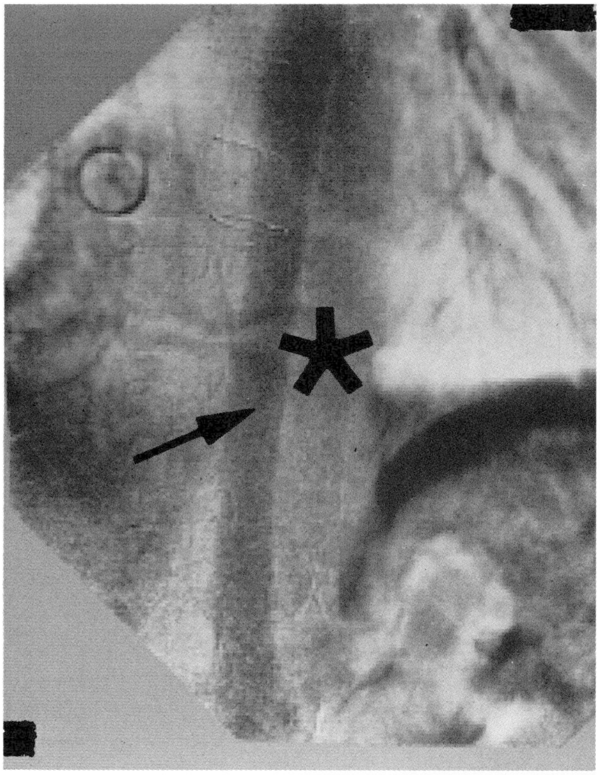 31

314, 315 Digital subtraction angiography in a patient with a dissecting aortic aneurysm. The true and false lumen can be clearly seen. The true lumen is more densely opacified by contrast (arrowed) and the false lumen is wider and less densely opacified (starred).

Cerebral vascular disease

Epidemiological studies have shown that all grades of hypertension are a major risk factor for the development of cerebral ischaemia, both stroke and transient ischaemic attacks. As well as hypertension causing atheroma of the intra- and extra-cranial arteries, it also predisposes to intra-cranial haemorrhage from aneurysm formation and rupture.

316

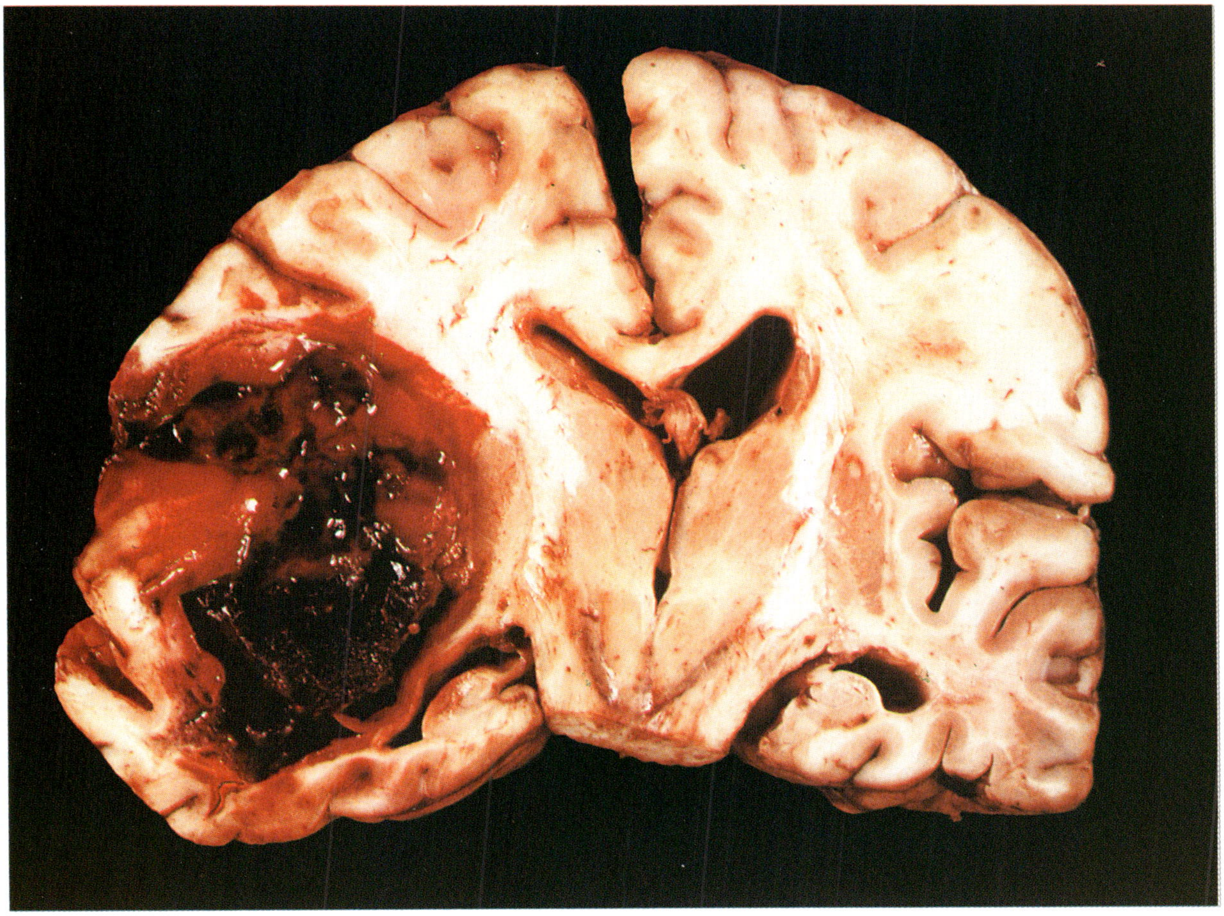

316 Coronal section through the brain showing a large haemorrhagic infarct.

317
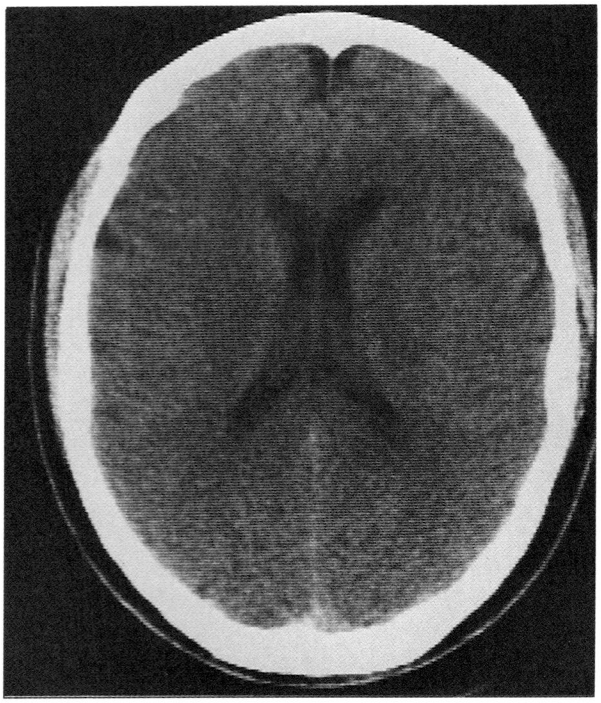

318
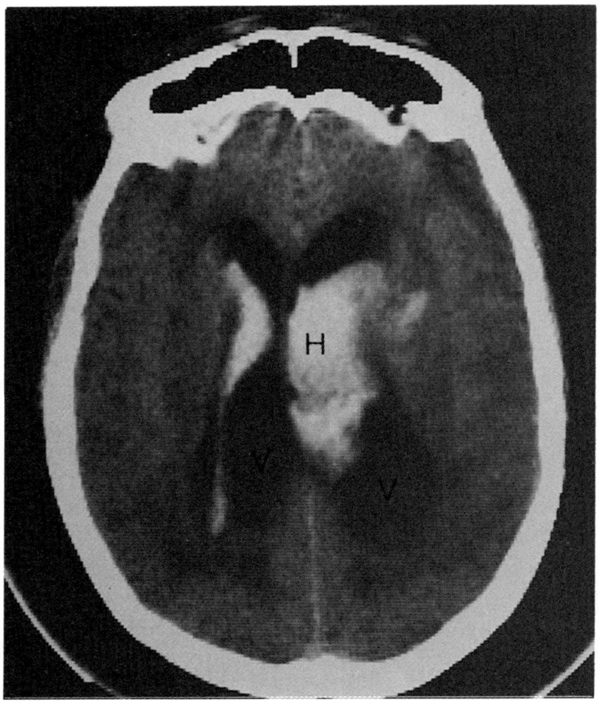

319
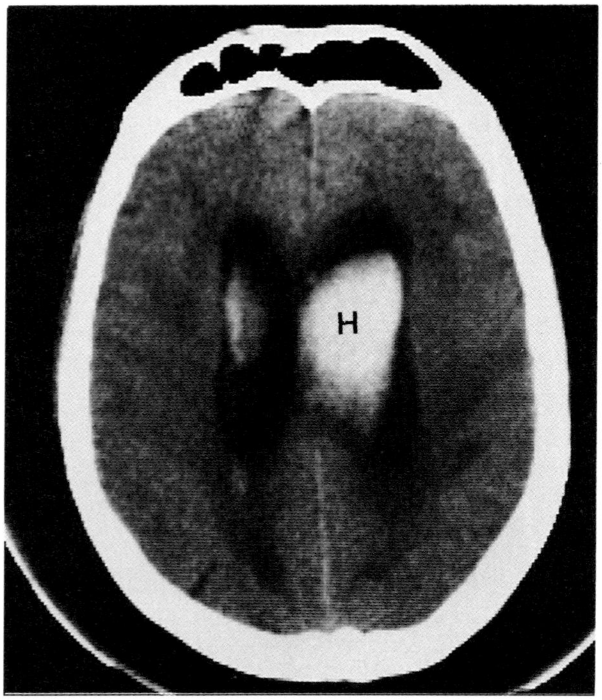

320
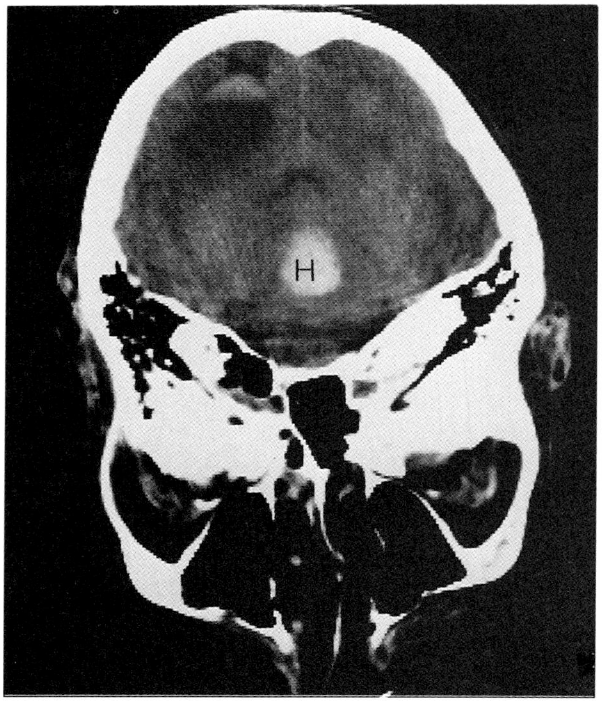

317–320 CT scans (transverse sections) through the head in cerebral vascular disease. **317** demonstrates a normal scan for comparison. Blood is seen within the substance of the brain and in particular within the lateral ventricle (**318**, H). Both ventricles (V) are dilated due to a previous intracerebral bleed (**319**). In **320**, a section more caudally taken shows the haemorrhage extending into the third ventricle.

321 CT scan showing cerebral haemorrhage (H) within the substance of the brain.

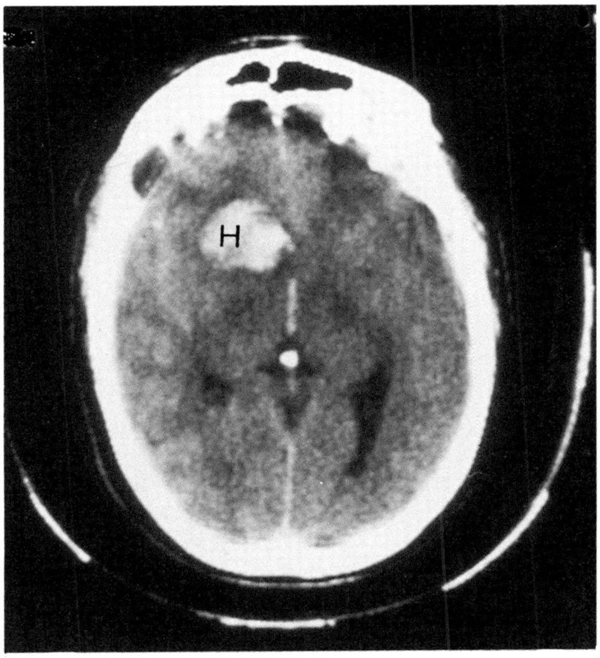

321

322

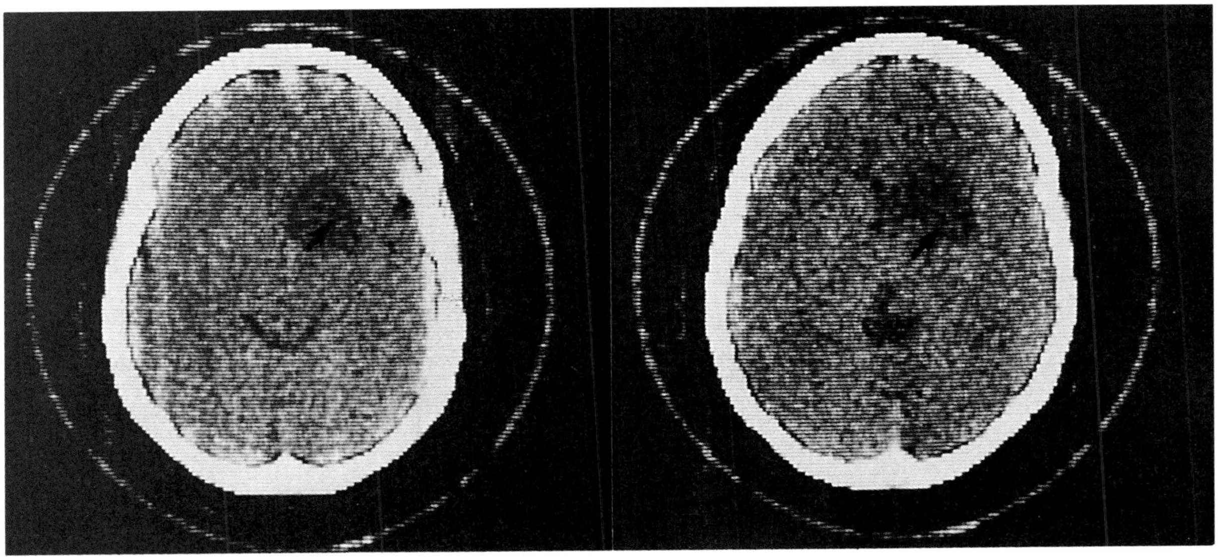

322 Transverse CT sections of a hypertensive patient who has suffered a stroke. A large infarct is seen (arrowed).

323

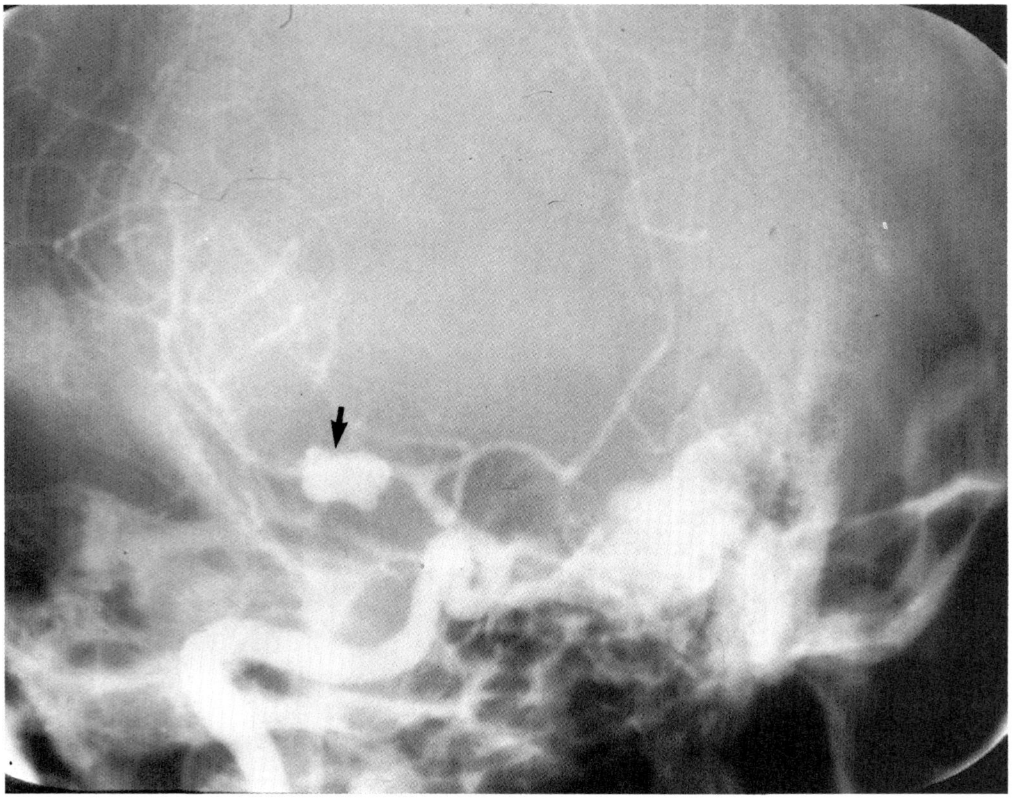

323 Selective carotid angiography showing an aneurysm (arrow) of the middle cerebral artery. Such aneurysms may lead to the type of intracranial haemorrhage seen in **322**.

324

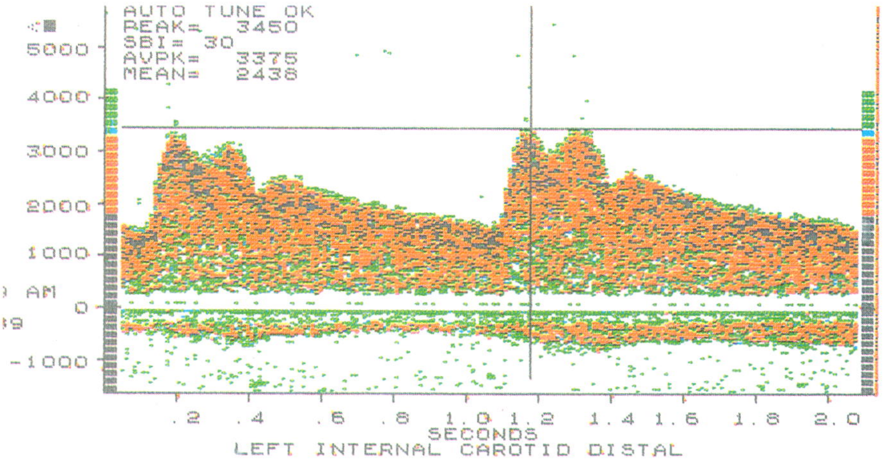

325

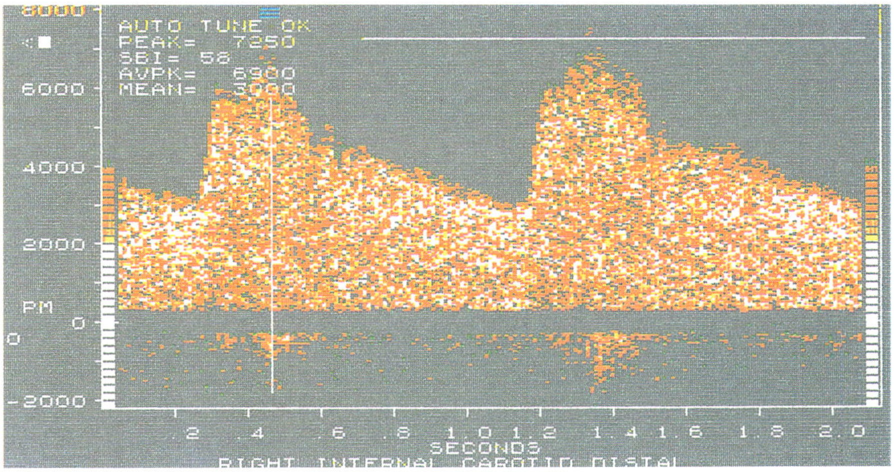

326

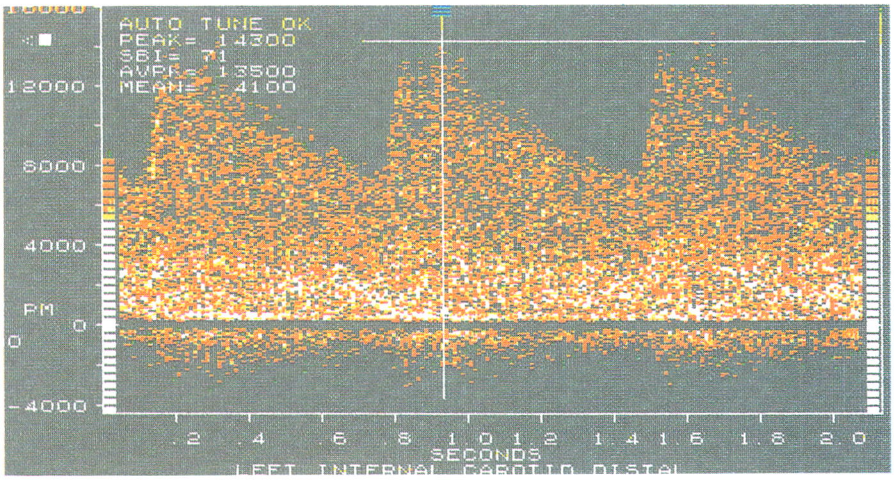

324–326 Doppler studies of the internal carotid arteries showing normal spectral waveforms (**324**), turbulence and increased peak velocity and reduced window in mild stenosis (**325**), and high peak velocity and absent window in severe stenosis (**326**).

327

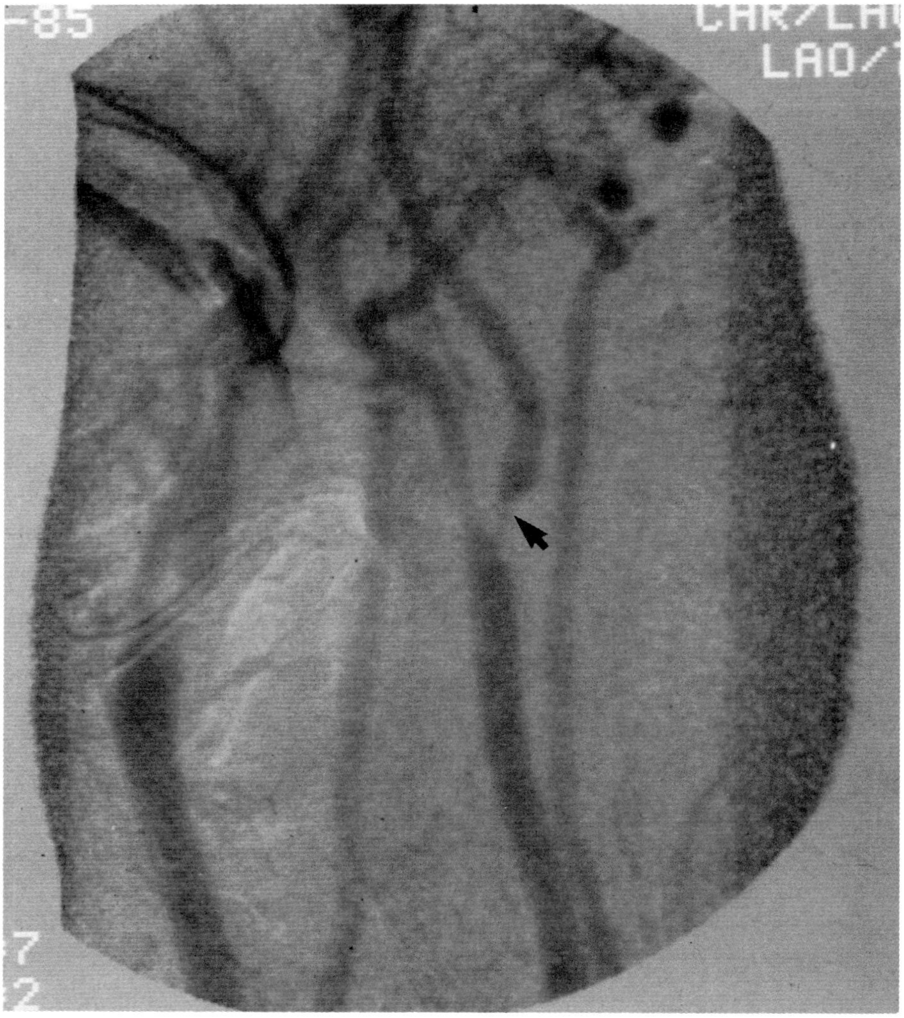

327 Digital subtraction angiogram showing a significant stenosis in the left internal carotid artery.

Principles of treatment of hypertension

The aim of treatment of hypertension is to reduce blood pressure to approaching the normal range. As the majority of patients are asymptomatic, blood pressure reduction needs to be carried out without significant side effects. In this section we will consider management of the hypertensive patient and the mechanisms of drug action, but not specific agents, as this is a rapidly evolving field with the development of new drugs and classes of drugs.

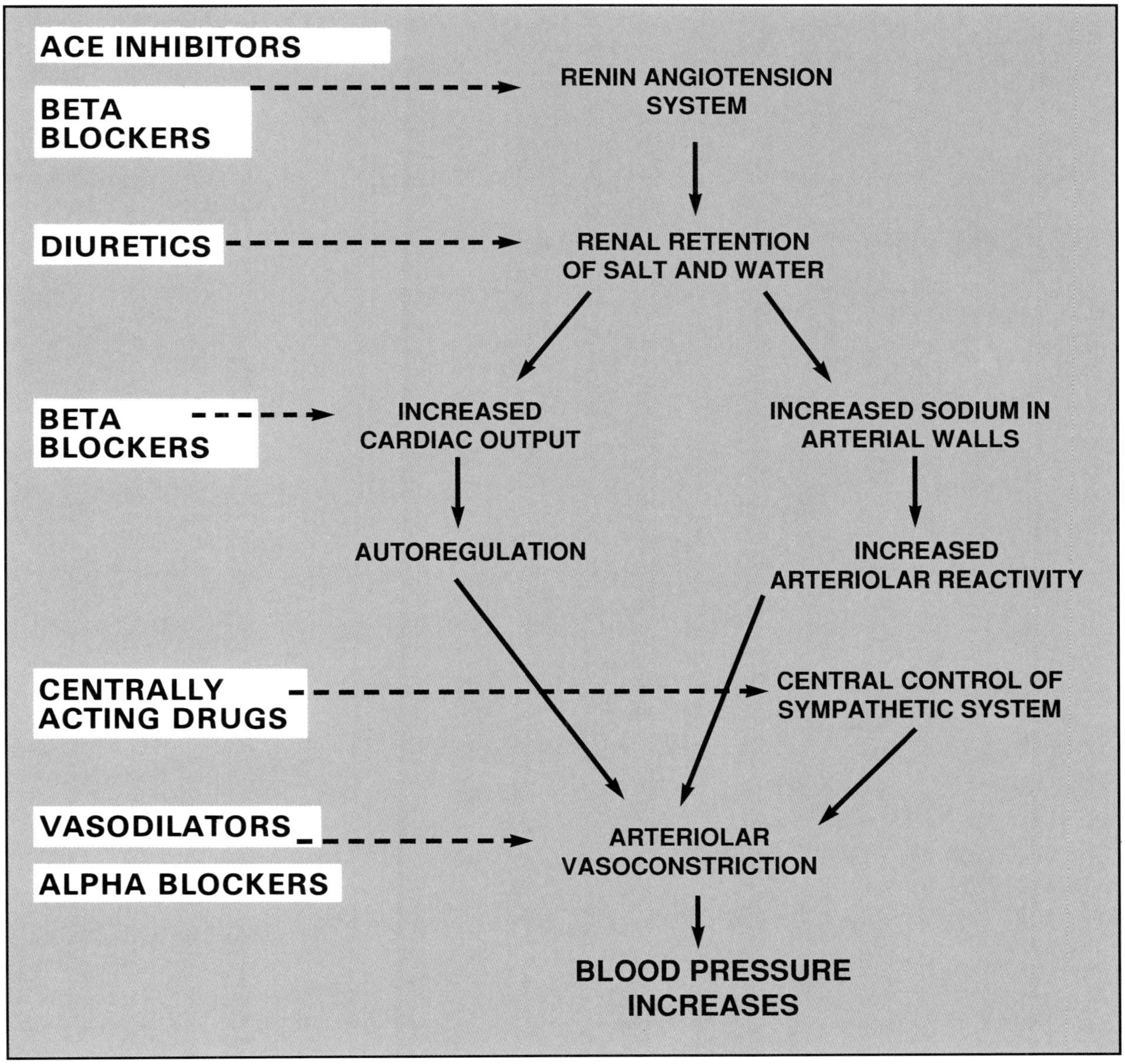

328

328 A schematic representation of the pathophysiological mechanisms that occur in the development of hypertension. The sites of action of the major classes of antihypertensive drugs are shown.

329

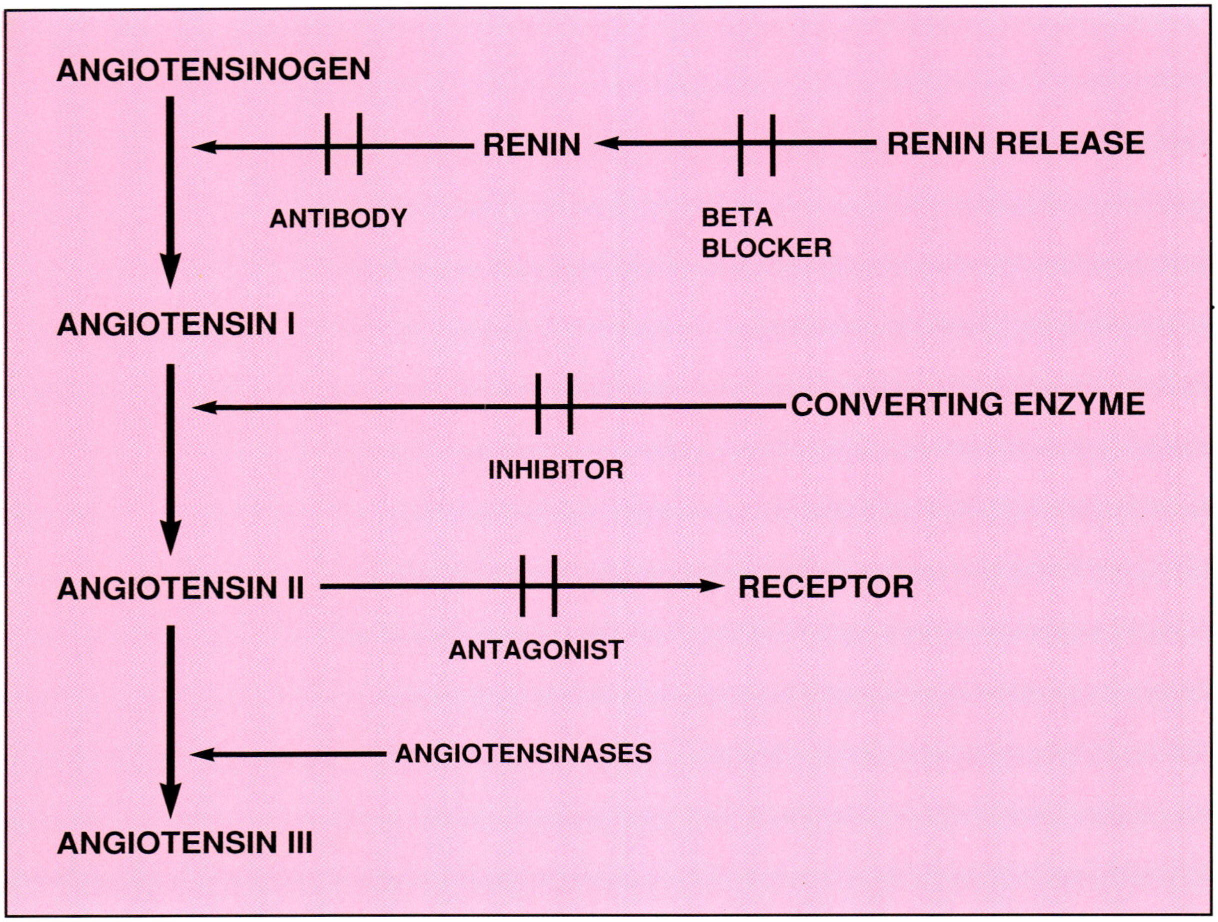

329 A schematic representation of the renin angiotensin system. The sites of action of betablockers and converting enzyme inhibitors are shown. Angiotensin is released in the liver, and renin from the kidney.

330

DRUG CLASS	CARDIAC OUTPUT	PERIPHERAL RESISTANCE	BLOOD VOLUME	PLASMA RENIN
DIURETICS	↔	↓	↓	↓
ALPHA BLOCKERS	↔↓	↔↓	↓	↓
BETA BLOCKERS	↓	↑	↔	↓
VASO-DILATORS	↑	↓	↑	↑

330 The major classes of antihypertensive drugs reduce arterial blood pressure by a number of different mechanisms. The effect of each of these drug classes is shown on cardiac output, peripheral vascular resistance of blood volume and plasma renin concentrate. Which of these mechanisms is most advantageous remains unclear.

331

TREATMENT	MECHANISM	INTERVENTION	BP REDUCTION
SALT RESTRICTION	REDUCED INTRA-VASCULAR VOLUME REDUCED VESSEL WALL SODIUM	DIETARY ADVICE Na INTAKE 100 mmol/DAY	8–15 mmHg SYSTOLIC 5–8 mmHg DIASTOLIC
RELAXATION	REDUCED SYMPATHETIC ACTIVITY	RELAXATION TECHNIQUES	9–27 mmHg SYSTOLIC 4–16 mmHg DIASTOLIC
WEIGHT LOSS	REDUCED SYMPATHETIC ACTIVITY REDUCED SODIUM INTAKE	DIET EXERCISE	9–27 mmHg MEAN
EXERCISE	REDUCED PERIPHERAL RESISTANCE WEIGHT LOSS	AEROBIC EXERCISE PROGRAMME	6–13 mmHg SYSTOLIC 9–12 mmHg DIASTOLIC

331 Various non-pharmacological methods have been tried to reduce blood pressure. Weight restriction, relaxation, weight loss and exercise all have a small effect on reducing blood pressure. In a patient with only mild hypertension, such measures may be effective alone. In a more severely hypertensive patient the use of non-pharmacological methods may occasionally reduce the need for drugs or achieve better blood pressure control. For these non-pharmacological methods to be effective, rigorous adherence to the regimens is necessary, and many patients find this difficult to maintain.

332

CAUSES OF FAILURE OF TREATMENT

1. LACK OF ADHERENCE TO REGIME
2. DRUG EFFECTIVENESS REDUCED BY
   a. INADEQUATE DOSES
   b. EXCESSIVE SALT
   c. DRUG INTERACTION
3. "OFFICE" HYPERTENSION
4. PRESSOR MECHANISM INTERFERING WITH DRUGS
   a. RELATED TO PRIMARY DISEASE e.g. PHAEOCHROMOCYTOMA
   b. COMPENSATORY MECHANISM e.g. SECONDARY ALDOSTERONISM
5. COMPLICATION OF LONG STANDING HYPERTENSION
   a. NEPHROSCLEROSIS
   b. LOSS OF AORTIC DISTENSIBILITY

332 The causes of failure of antihypertensive treatment are various. The most common is failure to adhere to the medication or other methods which have been employed. Many patients are hypertensive when examined in a clinic but ambulatory or home blood pressure recordings show good blood pressure control. Occasionally a pressor mechanism may interfere with the action of drugs, such as in phaeochromocytoma or the compensatory mechanisms occurring with secondary aldosteronism. Occasionally, in the long-standing hypertensive patient, renal or arterial abnormalities may interfere with the effectiveness of medication in reducing blood pressure.

References

Data for **2** and **12–46** were taken from the following references:

Fig.

2 Australian National Blood Pressure Study Management Committee. The Australian therapeutic trial in mild hypertension. *Lancet,* **1**, 1261:1980.

Hamilton M, Thompson EN, Wisnewski TKM. The role of blood pressure control in preventing the complications of hypertension. *Lancet,* **1**, 235:1964.

Medical Research Council Working Party. MRC trial of treatment of mild hypertension: principal results. *Br. Med. J.,* **291**, 97:1985.

Veterans Administrative Cooperative Group. Effects of treatment on the morbidity of hypertension: results in patients with diastolic blood pressures averaging 115 through 129 mmHg. *J. Am. Med. Soc.,* **202**, 1028:1967.

Veterans Administrative Cooperative Group. Effects of treatment on the morbidity of hypertension: results in patients with diastolic blood pressures averaging 90 through 114 mmHg. *J. Am. Med. Soc.,* **213**, 1143:1970.

12, 15 Voors AW, Weber LS, Berenson A. Relationship of blood pressure levels to height and weight in children. *Cardiovasc. Med.,* **3**, 911:1978.

13, 14 Whelton PK. Blood pressure in adults and the elderly, in *Handbook of Hypertension,* Vol. 6, Bulpitt CJ (ed), Elsevier, 1985.

16 Kannel WB. Host and environmental determinants in hypertension, in *Epidemiology of Arterial Blood Pressure,* Kesteloot H and Joosens JV (eds), Martinus Nijhoff, 1980.

17 Stamler J, Berkson DM, Dyer A, Lepper MH, Lindberg HA, Paul O, McKeon H, Rhomberg P, Schoenberger JA, Shekelle RB, Stamler R. Relationship of multiple variables to blood pressure, in *Epidemiology and Control of Hypertension,* Paul O (ed), Stratton, 1975.

18, 19 Beaglehole R, Salmond CE, Hooper A, Prior IAM. Blood pressure and social interaction in Tokelan migrants in New Zealand. *J. Chronic Dis.,* **30**, 803:1977.

20 Cassel JH. Studies in hypertension in migrants, in *Epidemiology and Control of Hypertension,* Paul O (ed), Stratton, 1975.

21 Tyroler HA, Heyden S, Hames CG. Weight and hypertension: Evans County studies of blacks and whites, in *Epidemiology and Control of Hypertension,* Paul O (ed), Stratton, 1975.

22 Marmot MG, Rose G, Shipley M, Hamilton PJS. Employment grade and coronary heart disease in British Civil Servants. *J. Epidemiol. Commun. Health,* **32**, 244:1978.

23 Komachi Y, Shimamoto T. Salt intake and its relationship to blood pressure in Japan past and present, in *Epidemiology of Arterial Blood Pressure,* Kesteloot H and Joosens JV (eds), Martinus Nijhoff, 1980.

24 Shaper AG, Popock SJ, Walker M, Cohen NM, Wale CJ, Thompson AG. British Regional Heart Study: cardiovascular risk factors in middle-aged men in 24 towns. *Br. Med. J.,* **283**, 179:1982.

25 Patel C, Marmot MG, Terry DJ. Controlled trial of biofeedback-aided behavioral methods in reducing mild hypertension. *Br. Med. J.,* **282**, 2005:1981.

26 Shurtleff D. Some characteristics related to the incidence of cardiovascular disease and death: Framingham Study, 18 year follow up, in *An Epidemiological Investigation of Cardiovascular Disease: The Framingham Study,* Kannel WB, Gordon T (eds), DHEW Publication No (NIH) 74–599.

27, 28 Bulpitt CJ. The prognosis of essential hypertension, in *Handbook of Hypertension,* Vol. 6, Bulpitt CJ (ed), Elsevier, 1985.

29–31 Dawber TR. *The Framingham Study: The Epidemiology of Atherosclerotic Disease,* Harvard University Press, 1980.

32, 33 Shaper AG, Pocock SJ, Walker M, Phillips AN, Whitehead TP, McFarlane PW. Risk factors for ischaemic heart disease: the prospective phase of the British Regional Heart Study. *J. Edpidemiol. Commun. Health,* **39**, 197:1985.

34–36 Kannel WB, Sorlie P. Hypertension in Framingham, in *Edpidemiology and Control of Hypertension,* Paul O (ed), Stratton, 1975.

37 Marmot MG. Diet, hypertension and stroke, in *Nutrition and Health,* Tuner MR (ed), MTP, 1982.

38 Assmann G, Schulte H. The prospective cardiovascular Münster (PROCAM) study: prevalence of hyperlipidemia in persons with hypertension and/or diabetes mellitus and the relationship to coronary heart disease. *Am. Heart J.,* **116**, 1713:1988.

39 Castelli WP. Epidemiology of coronary heart disease – the Framingham Study. *Am. J. Med.,* **76**, 4:1984.

40 See **2**, Veterans Administrative Cooperative Group, 1970.

41–46 Amery A, Birkenhager W, Brixko P. Mortality and morbidity results from the European Working Party on High Blood Pressure in the Elderly trial. *Lancet,* **i**, 1349:1985.

Collins R, Peto R, McMahon S, Hebert P, Fiebach NH, Eberlein KA, Godwin J, Qizilbash N, Taylor JO, Hennekens CH. Blood pressure, stroke and coronary heart disease. Part 2, short term reductions in blood pressure: overview of randomised drug trials in their epidemiological context. *Lancet,* **335**, 827:1990.

Coope J, Warrender TS. Randomised trial of treatment of hypertension in the elderly in primary care. *Br. Med. J.,* **293**, 1145:1986.

Hypertension Detection and Follow-up Program Cooperative Group. Five year findings of the Hypertension Detection and Follow-up Program I. Reduction in mortality among persons with high blood pressure including mild hypertension. *JAMA,* **242**, 2562:1979.

Hypertension Detection and Follow-up Program Cooperative Group. Five year findings of the Hypertension Detection and Follow-up Program II. Mortality by race, sex and age. *JAMA,* **242**, 2572:1979.

Index

B

C

D

E

F

G

H

I

J

K

O

P

Q

R

S

T

U

V

W